60 WAYS
TO KEEP YOUR
Brain Sharp

BONNIE BETH SPARRMAN, BSN

HARVEST HOUSE PUBLISHERS
EUGENE, OREGON

Cover by Bryce Williamson

Cover image © chatchaisurakram / iStock

Back cover author photo © by Christopher Erickson

All oven temperatures are given in degrees Fahrenheit.

60 WAYS TO KEEP YOUR BRAIN SHARP

Copyright © 2018 by Bonnie Beth Sparrman
Published by Harvest House Publishers
Eugene, Oregon 97408
www.harvesthousepublishers.com

ISBN 978-0-7369-7209-3 (pbk.)
ISBN 978-0-7369-7210-9 (eBook)

Library of Congress Cataloging-in-Publication Data

Names: Sparrman, Bonnie Beth, author.
Title: 60 ways to keep your brain sharp / Bonnie Beth Sparrman.
Other titles: Sixty ways to keep your brain sharp
Description: Eugene, Oregon : Harvest House Publishers, [2018]
Identifiers: LCCN 2017035967 (print) | LCCN 2017036347 (ebook) | ISBN 9780736972109 (ebook) | ISBN 9780736972093 (pbk.)
Subjects: LCSH: Brain--Aging--Prevention. | Brain--Care and hygiene. | Brain--Diseases--Nutritional aspects. | Mental health. | Self-care, Health.
Classification: LCC QP376 (ebook) | LCC QP376 .S737 2018 (print) | DDC 612.8/2--dc23
LC record available at https://lccn.loc.gov/2017035967

For my husband, Eric,
whose constant love is my delight,
and for my father, Bendt Bladel,
whose perseverance is my inspiration.

Acknowledgments

Writing is a funny thing; it is done mostly in isolation but not without a lot of help from others. I have been abundantly blessed by many who have generously offered inspiration, ideas, prayers, and encouragement. First of all, I'm extremely grateful for the sage advice of author and editor Todd Hafer. I owe many thanks to Todd for giving me this opportunity to write. Without his talent and trust, this book would not be. Also, I am thankful for Kim Moore, a seasoned editor, for her kindness and for her wise way with words.

I am also deeply indebted to my older friends who are stellar examples of vibrant brain health. First, I think of my dad, Bendt, who at 89 is sharp, athletic, persevering, and not afraid to learn new things. I am grateful for the way he lives, for his good genes, his enduring love, and for choosing a fabulous wife. He and my mother, Elaine, whom we lost to cancer way too early, looked beyond themselves with genuine interest in people of all ages.

Others who inspired this book include Stig Benson, Bonnie Abrahamson, Ken Vogel, Adaline Bjorkman, Harriet Lonergan, Ruth Petersen, Ginny Graham, Helen Pattie, Ingrid Bergstrom, Jack and Joan Streed, John and Mary Anderson, Bill and Jean Bristow, Dr. Wyatt and Nancy Moe, Marvin Bjorlin, Aunt Susann Gustafson, and my loving parents-in-law, Paul and Gunnie Sparrman. Thank you all for living long lives so beautifully.

Who could embark on a writing project without dear friends and family members to cheer and encourage? I owe tremendous gratitude to my wonderful children—Johanna, Bjorn, Karl-Jon, and Isa—and to my supportive siblings, Krissy, Gordy, Randy, Julie, Jon, Randi, Lisa, and Jim.

And what an enormous gift to have a covey of friends who lift me up along the way. I am especially thankful for Shelley Frew (my faithful confidante and pen pal for life), Lora "Gus" Plude, Åsa Linbro, Helena Folcker, Joey Nytes, Barbara and Steven Swanson, Jane Frasier, Sue Beck, Dr. Linda Solie, Joy Larson, Linda Peterson, Kristina Krafthefer, Molly Braley, Nancy Stark, Paige Vandegrift, Dr. Karen Tamte, Tim and Cyd Johnson, and Nancy Nordenson. Your help in practical ways, and in allowing your life stories to intersect with mine, thrills my heart and spurs me on.

Lastly, and most poignantly, God has blessed me through my ever-abiding husband, Eric. His love, patience, faithful prayers, technical skills, and coffee roasting abilities keep the journey light, exciting, and full of joy! It is my dream that together he and I will be riding our bikes to the bakery for decades to come. Honey, I owe you more than *pain au chocolat*!

Contents

Part Three: Intellectual Stimulation

Part Four: Social and Spiritual Stimulation

God Made Us Smart— Let's Stay That Way

From the vastness of the Milky Way to the grandeur of oceans and mountain ranges, and all the way down to the tiny legs of honeybees, God's handiwork is magnificent. Yet, as we contemplate the breadth of creation, it's not an exaggeration to say that the human brain is God's masterpiece. Consider this: Every movement, every heartfelt pang, and every wild idea originates in our body's mission-control center, the brain. This three-pound mass of firm jelly sitting between our ears is so important that God surrounded it with a protective, built-in helmet called the cranium.

As a nursing student, I was fascinated to discover that our miraculous brains are a forest of more than 100 billion nerve cells linked at more than 100 trillion points. Signals fly faster than the blink of an eye through this forest, forming the basis of memories, thoughts, and feelings. Within each person's gray matter lies the unique code that makes us who we are. Electrical impulses whiz through the labyrinth, determining our personality, temperament, and values, as well as our ability to see, move, hear, taste, smell, reason, create, believe, solve problems, and be in relationship with others. Without your amazing brain, you would not be *you*.

Because our brains make up the very essence of who we are, we need them to function well throughout our entire lifespan. We enter the world as helpless infants, dependent on others for our survival. Through love and nurturing care, we master baby skills and become toddlers who pull ourselves up to stand, walk, and then run circles around our parents' legs. We scamper through childhood, limbs elongating and minds growing. Then, for better or for worse, another metamorphosis takes place. Children become teenagers. Eventually, they grow into young adults. All the while, brains are developing on myriad levels.

Fluid intelligence, the ability to logically solve problems, develops with us. Crystalized intelligence, which lets us apply our knowledge and experience, also expands as we mature to adulthood. And then what happens to our capacity to think?

You might have heard devastating reports that brainpower peaks at 18 and, following that auspicious age, we suffer a depressing decline. This is not completely true. Thanks to a couple of bright MIT researchers, Hartshorne and Germine, who have studied the brain function of 50,000 participants, we now know that different cognitive skills peak at various points along life's journey.[1]

While it's true that our ability to *swiftly* process new information may peak around age 20, our short-term memory does not peak until 25. It remains very high until about 35. Even more encouraging is the discovery that our ability to evaluate other people's emotional states isn't optimal until we are in our forties or fifties. And crystalized intelligence, which gives us access to accumulated knowledge, peaks in our late sixties or early seventies. Especially for those who keep working and reading, vocabularies continue to expand, and we are able to build on previous knowledge. This is good news for all of us.

Joshua Hartshorne, one of the MIT study's authors (now doing post-doctoral research at MIT's Department of Brain and Cognitive Sciences), says, "At any given age, you're getting better at some things, you're getting worse at some other things, and you're at a plateau at some other things. There's probably not one age at which you're peak on most things, much less all of them."[2]

Still, it is no surprise to any of us that the more we use our intellect, the better our minds continue to function. For athletes who hope to improve their tennis game, practice on the court and staying in shape are necessary if they are to excel. The same is true for keeping our brains sharp. We need to stretch and flex intellectually if we are to have a nimble brain.

But keeping our minds in shape is not limited to mental calisthenics. We must also move our bodies, the machines that house and support our brains. Many studies point to the fact that people who exercise regularly, eat well, and maintain a healthy body weight are mentally sharper than their sedentary and overweight contemporaries. It is a proven fact that those who suffer from poorly managed chronic illnesses such as hypertension; diabetes; high cholesterol; and heart, kidney, and liver disease also lag behind mentally. And while sometimes these diseases pop up against all odds, without any fault of the person who becomes ill, they are often avoidable.

In addition to choosing a physically healthy lifestyle, staying connected with others is vital. Stimulating relationships, in which mutual caring and interesting interchange are natural parts of each day, promote good mental function. Conversely, lack of community, which leads to isolation and loneliness, does not do a brain or a soul any good.

In this book, we will explore ways to keep our brains sharp and functioning to their utmost, giving us high-quality lives for as long as possible. We will consider:

- Physical activity
- Nutrition
- Intellectually stimulating activities
- Social and spiritual connections

As we take steps to preserve and enhance brain function, we begin an exciting journey that will help us live more enjoyable and fulfilling lives. Being better stewards of God's greatest creation, our brain, will promote positive results for ourselves and for those we love most dearly. Increasing our capacity to think is a brilliant investment in the present as well as the future.

Part One

Physical Activity and Related Preventive Measures

At the Beach, Pondering Midlife Fitness

Early in the morning, before everyone at the beach house wakes up, I silently climb out the bedroom window and scamper down a path to the lake, trying in vain to avoid acorns and stones with my bare feet. In the crook of my arm are a towel, a few books, and a pen. From my spot on the dune, between tufts of beach grass, the sound of waves soothes and invigorates me. I read, write, and stretch. Then I go for a run before diving into the surf. The beach may seem a strange setting for thoughts on brain health, but hang with me.

This beach, on the eastern shore of Lake Michigan, has been home to me more than anywhere else. It was a constant in my life even during years of transiency. It's where I learned to walk, swim, and tumble. The same is true for my children. It is also where we watched grandparents grow old, and more recently, my dad. So when summer comes, it's important for my family to return to the dunes, sit on the sand, and review where we've been, as well as consider where we are right now and contemplate dreams for the future.

For better or for worse, my husband and I dangle from the last car of the baby boomer train. This means we were born just in time to eat a plethora of processed foods and watch *The Wonderful World of Disney* on Sunday nights. In the 1960s, most homes had a TV, which told us what to purchase—from margarine to processed cereals. On the bright side, as children we enjoyed freedom, roaming vast blocks of neighborhoods, playing in creek beds, and climbing trees while clutching bags of penny candy.

Today, we baby boomers have come of age. And along with our maturity come not only all kinds of blessings, but also fears about the future. If I have felt unprepared for any stage of life, this middle-age segment is it. Though I watched my mom and dad diligently care for their aging parents, I didn't understand the gravity of their efforts. Now that it's our turn to help dads and moms navigate their eighties (and, soon, nineties), we see more clearly the difficulties that come with old age. As we hold the car door and slowly help parents in or out, we realize, *"Yikes, we're next!"*

It comes as no surprise that baby boomers' greatest concerns upon retirement are for financial security and retaining our mental marbles.[1] Considering what it costs to care for a person with dementia, these concerns are closely intertwined.

From my sandy perch on the dune, my mind's eye turns to my grandfather, a hardworking electrician whose foresight led our family to this beach in the 1940s. Harold stood just about five feet seven, but he was strong of body, lean, and industrious.

When I was a teenager and he was in his seventies, I remember him missing the turn-off to our favorite hardware store. I was alarmed, but my grandma had already been noting lapses like this. At the time, I knew nothing about dementia. I didn't understand what was happening to my intelligent grandpa, a guy who could fix anything.

Today, as I read the literature about dementia, I find it makes no sense that my grandfather's mind would cloud over, even to the point of failing to recognize his own family members. Yes, his diet was so-so, but he was never overweight. He never smoked, and he never drank anything stronger than coffee. He stayed socially engaged, chauffeuring dozens of widows to various appointments and fixing their broken clocks and toasters.

He exercised regularly. He walked up and down hills to get the mail. He cut down trees with my Uncle Ephraim. The two of them sang together too, beautiful duets in church. Ephraim sang baritone, and Grandpa carried the tenor part with ease.

The doctor called Grandpa Harold's condition "hardening of the arteries." The oxygen-rich blood wasn't getting to all the places in Grandpa's brain. So, bit by bit, his brain was shutting down. It was painful to watch, especially for Gram, who never fully understood that Grandpa had no control over the matter. "Being in our right mind" isn't always a choice. We don't get to pick which part of us goes haywire first. And this is why we baby boomers are biting our nails.

But we *can* do more than nibble our digits. As science produces studies on nutrition, exercise, brain games, and many methods to keep us thinking, we can take that knowledge and put it to good use. Though there is not yet a cure for Alzheimer's disease, we do know that certain behaviors help stave it off.

From my beach towel, as I see a lot of humanity walk past, I'm reminded that we do have some control over our size. Body mass index (BMI) is a number that provides a benchmark for how we are doing with our weight. BMI factors in our height relative to our weight. Our BMI number places us into one of four categories: underweight, normal, overweight, or obese. I want to point out that this number does *not* reflect a person's self-worth.

The easiest way to find your BMI is to use an online BMI calculator. Pop in your height and weight and in a second you'll know your BMI. If your number lands in the overweight or obese range, you are not alone. More than two-thirds of American adults fall into these categories, with 28 percent weighing in as obese.

Statistically speaking, being overweight or obese at age 50 increases the risk of dementia later in life, including Alzheimer's disease.[2] Plus, the higher the BMI, the sooner dementia may affect one's brain.

Obviously, it's not possible to alter genetic factors connected to dementia, but working toward a healthier BMI is within our reach. In the next few chapters we'll look at various ways to burn calories through exercise. And moving our bodies will move our BMIs to a healthier place.

Take a Hike

Stig is a wonderful older athlete whose trim physique and healthy countenance belie his 86 years. Raised on a dairy farm in southern Sweden, Stig grew up in pristine nature. Rolling hills, plenty of water, and pine forests surrounded his home, beckoning him to wander wooded paths, foraging for mushrooms and wild berries. Stig is the most aptly named person I know, because his name, pronounced *Steeg* in Swedish, means "pathway or wanderer." When his parents chose this name for the first of their seven children, I wonder if they knew how perfectly it would fit him his entire life.

Stig has always loved the forest. He took to the woods on foot during sunny Swedish summers, and on cross-country skis in the winter. Skiing, hiking, and bike riding were his modes of transportation as he grew into a strong young man. Out in the forest, he traversed many miles, hunting deer and moose. This helped his parents put meat on the table for their large family.

Stig was not only an adventurer in nature; he also ventured out to start a career. As the firstborn, he was to inherit the family farm. But Stig had a mind for engineering, not farming. So he took a different path. After studying engineering in college, he landed a job at SAAB, where he worked in the stress calculation department for supersonic jets. One day, he received an invitation to work in his uncle's construction company across the ocean in Chicago. After much contemplation, the 26-year-old left Sweden and immigrated to the United States. He worked hard in the company. A couple of years later, he married a Swedish beauty who was also new to America. Stig and Ingrid settled into suburban life near Chicago, where they raised four children, one of whom became my childhood friend.

It is not hard to imagine that life in a Chicago suburb is extremely different from life in rural Sweden. For a guy who leapt over fences and ran along the banks of deep blue lakes and timber roads, Chicago's suburban square blocks of houses must have felt restrictive. Forest preserves were a pathetic replacement for the vast woods that Stig had known. Still, he acclimated well to American life while holding on to a few Swedish ways. Much to the embarrassment of his kids, Stig trained for cross-country ski races by roller-skiing around town. He was the only person we knew to "ski" past our house on a clear October day. And he hiked the paths along Salt Creek in Fullersburg, the closest thing our neighborhood had to deep woods.

Now in retirement, Stig and Ingrid spend winters in Green Valley, Arizona, where Stig is an avid member of a hiking club. Every Thursday, Ingrid packs a hearty lunch, and Stig takes off to meet his buddies to hike in the mountains. With trekking poles in hand and solid boots on their feet, the hikers spend the entire day traversing the beautiful hillsides that surround Green Valley and Tucson. They hike for fun, a group of 200 or more who are doubly blessed by their efforts.

Why doubly blessed? Like Stig, these happy wanderers enjoy the simple act of hiking. But do they know they are promoting brain health as they hike? Research at several universities has revealed great benefits to hiking—benefits beyond the obvious. Yes, hiking is good for cardiorespiratory health, and it promotes strong muscle tone. And, of course, it burns calories, (400 to 700 per hour), which helps decrease the risk of diabetes. But, you might ask, couldn't these benefits be gained in a gym?

Here's where the "wow factor" enters the picture. Scientists have recently discovered that hiking in a natural setting lowers rumination (focusing on negative or distressing thoughts), boosts creative thinking, and decreases the risk of depression and the negative symptoms of attention deficit hyperactivity disorder (ADHD).[1] Plus, amazingly, it promotes healing from cancer by lessening the oxidative process in our blood.

Let's start with rumination, that exhausting tendency to replay negative, embarrassing, or shameful memories over and over. When we ruminate, we increase blood flow to the part of our brains that is linked to mental illness. Rumination is a negative pull on our psyche, and it often precedes depression and anxiety. In a Stanford study, a group of people was sent out to hike for 90 minutes. Half of them hiked in an urban area, while half enjoyed a peaceful, natural setting. Upon returning from their trek, only those who took the nature hike were found, by MRI and by questionnaire, to have enjoyed a calming, nonruminating experience. Those who walked in a busy urban area experienced more negative thought processes. Our brains respond more positively as we hike in nature.[2]

Another study focused on oxidative effects on long-distance hikers. One way our bodies protect themselves is via a high antioxidative capacity. As you may know, antioxidants protect our bodies from harmful molecules called free radicals. Our antioxidative defenses prevent cancer cells from going nuts and starting trouble in our bodies. A group of German researchers discovered that people who hike in nature have better antioxidative defenses than their peers, supporting the idea that hiking can help prevent cancer.[3] I'll hike to that!

And if warding off depression and cancer isn't enough reason to push us out the door for a good hike in the woods, let's consider what a nature walk does for those who suffer with ADHD. Researchers at the University of Illinois found that children with ADHD (and who exhibit impulsivity and distractibility) concentrate and control themselves much better after hiking in a natural setting. These researchers took three groups of children outside for walks. One group hiked in a noisy urban setting, one in a semi-green space, and the last in a "very green" area. They found that the more natural the hiking environment, the more the kids could concentrate on mental tasks afterward.[4]

With so many great reasons to grab our hiking shoes and hit the trails, how nice that hiking is relatively easy to begin. All you need are a comfortable pair of walking shoes, a water bottle, and perhaps a set of trekking poles to take some pressure off the knees. Many parks provide trail maps to keep you on track. And like Stig, you might find a group of other hikers and build friendships along the way. Even in urban settings, parks provide wonderful places to walk—places that give our minds a break, refreshing us for the challenges of the day. While extremely few of us have a name that means "pathway," all of us can benefit from a mind-healing hike in the woods or a walk in the park.

Go Jump in the Lake

When my family vacations with my dad, inevitably someone will tell him, "Go jump in the lake." No one means any disrespect. We all understand that Papa is much cheerier after a good swim. At 89, my dad still swims like a fish. I believe his love of water began as a boy growing up on Chicago's South Side in a home where central heat was a luxury and air conditioning was out of the question. All summer long, he and his buddies made their way to the beaches along Lake Michigan. There they found relief from the scorching heat and humidity that hung over Chicago like pea soup. They spent hours in the lake, daring each other to swim out past the sand bar, strengthening their ability day by day.

At 16, my dad was thrilled to get a job lifeguarding on Jackson Beach. From his lifeguard stand he could check out the girls; and on his breaks, he could plunge into the waves to cool off.

Being daredevils abounding with youthful invincibility, my dad and a few of his pals were known to swim out to Chicago's 68th Street water-intake crib, 2.3 miles offshore. Any sensible mother would consider this highly dangerous—and so did the coast guard. When some "Coasties" discovered the boys swimming a mile offshore, they delivered a serious scolding. My dad, however, enjoyed the long-distance swims and didn't give up easily. The second time the coast guard hauled him out of the water and into a lifeboat, an officer gave him a long look and, shaking his head, exclaimed, "Not *you* again!" This put an end to Dad's audacious swims, because he wanted keep his job as a lifeguard.

All that to say, without swimming lessons or even a high school with a swim team, my father has been a champion swimmer his entire life. When I was a kid, I swam next to him for hours and hours, lap after lap, father and daughter enjoying the water together. He taught me to keep stroking through tired lulls, pushing on to a second wind. As an adult, he introduced me to former Olympians and ordinary guys with whom he swims early on summer mornings. Now as an octogenarian who still loves to swim, he remains a fixture at his local pool, making waves with his favorite stroke, the butterfly. A few months ago, we swam together, and he clicked off a mile and a half with graceful ease. The only additions to his routine are a pair of flippers, a pull buoy, and sometimes a snorkel.

I know not everyone enjoys the water. I know people who hate to swim, and some who have no idea how it's done. Plenty of people are afraid of water and avoid any that is deeper than their bathtub. But exercising in water is incredibly good for us physically, and it's surprisingly positive for us mentally. Even if you are a nonswimmer, listen to what the National Institutes of Health says about exercising in water. The organization reports that blood flow to the brain is increased when a person is submerged in water to the level of his or her heart.[1]

Doing water aerobics or merely walking in a pool of chest-deep water improves cerebrovascular perfusion, or flow of vital fluids through our circulatory systems. One doesn't have to actually swim to reap the benefit of increased blood flow to the brain, which helps improve memory, mental clarity, mood, and the ability to focus.

Moreover, swimming and other aquatic exercise help decrease depression. As brain chemicals are stimulated, our mood is elevated and our general outlook brightens. A study at the University of Washington sports concussion program revealed that after 30 days of swimming, rats were happier and seemed less likely to experience panic. This may be partially due to the rhythmic stroking and regular breathing that accompany swimming or working out in water. It's much like the tension-reducing effects of meditative deep breathing.

Another way swimming boosts memory is through neurogenesis (the birth of new neurons) in the hippocampus, the brain's memory center. With a greater supply of oxygen going to the brain, the hippocampus will grow, and its ability to remember grows with it. It's easy to imagine that as a swimmer breathes deeply, the chest expands and the brain's hippocampus is the lucky recipient of a good supply of oxygen. This results in an improved memory.

If these benefits are not enough, you'll be interested to know that swimming also enhances visual motor skills, which, in turn, make learning easier. During swimming, the cross-pattern motion strengthens the development of the corpus callosum, the part of the brain that connects the left and right hemispheres. As these hemispheres are better connected and all four lobes of the brain are activated, we learn better.

In a 2012 study, researchers discovered that children who learned to swim early in life were better coordinated and reached developmental milestones more quickly. They exhibited better visual motor skills, such as cutting paper, coloring, drawing, and solving mathematical problems.

Last, I must mention the most obvious benefit of aquatic exercise. In the water, our muscles are toned and strengthened, while joints are protected by the shock-absorbing benefit of the water. Swimming is a great way to get in shape. It's easy to notice swimmers' sleek physiques, but who knew that being in water is also wonderful for the brain?

In our family we say, "Keep swimming, Papa," and I'll add "and everyone else who wishes to enhance memory, mood, and the ability to learn." The peaceful expression on the faces of people sauntering out of the pool is testimony enough to the benefits of swimming.

DID YOU KNOW?

- No one really cares what you look like in a bathing suit! Everyone else is too worried about his or her own physique to care about yours.
- When you go to the pool, a nice big thirsty towel is a great comfort.
- You can't help making friends at the pool.
- A person who weighs 150 pounds will burn about 500 calories in an hour of swimming.

Walk It Off

Our favorite comedian, who skillfully takes us from laugher to tears, performs a wonderful vignette where his father's cure for any of his son's pain (a twisted ankle, stomach ache, or blue mood) is *"Walk it off!"* Throughout the son's life, he is admonished over and over by these three words, words that don't sound all that comforting, especially while dealing with a bulging appendix. (True story!)

Eventually the tables turn when the son receives a call from his mom. She reports that Dad, now an old man, took a terrible fall from an apple tree and shattered his pelvis. She puts Dad on the phone, and the son hears the pain in his father's voice. Can you guess the punch line? Can you hear the audience laughing hysterically? The son makes a desperate attempt to resist uttering those three trusty words. But, thanks to his father, they are etched indelibly in his mind, ready to be spoken when pain strikes. He listens to his dad's report of the accident, and, being the jokester that he is, lovingly says, "Dad, you just need to...*walk it off*!"

During the explosion of applause that closes the scene, I find myself splitting a gut at the performer and also at myself. As good drama does, this scene uncovers truths about our own humanity. More personally, it points out my tendency to say to anyone not feeling well, "You just need more exercise and more water." This seems to work wonders for me. Why wouldn't it work for everyone else?

At the risk of sounding as unsympathetic as that old father, a lot of truth is in the assertion that we probably *do* need more exercise. For most people, the least expensive and easiest-access exercise is walking. Yes, let's get our buns off the couch, put on some comfortable shoes, and head out the door. Okay, on a day when it's pouring rain or sleeting sideways, it's not that simple. But there are malls; indoor tracks; and hallways of apartment buildings, office buildings, and churches where we can roam. A gaggle of walkers frequents our local Target store. Others like to traverse the corridors of our church.

I should note that here in Minnesota, the walking and cycling trail through the woods near our house is heavily used, even in the winter. The locals here are *hearty.*

We might think that plain walking can't be all that noteworthy in this world of Lycra-clad marathon runners and triathletes. But it is! A controlled research study led by a psychologist at the University of Pittsburgh offers results that encourage us to grab our walking shoes and go.

In the study, 120 seniors were divided into 2 groups. The first 60 seniors did stretching and yoga-type exercises for 40 minutes, 3 times a week. The other 60 participants walked on a track for the same amount of time. The results showed that the walkers experienced a 2 percent increase in the size of the hippocampus, the brain's short-term memory center.[1] We know that the hippocampus tends to shrink as we age, and the three days each week of walking negated that shrinkage.

By the way, the hippocampus is destroyed when a person has Alzheimer's, so these findings are significant. Also, the study showed that both the walkers and the stretchers performed better on spatial memory tests, which means they were more adept at remembering patterns. Yet only the walkers improved their aerobic capacity, which goes hand-in-hand with better blood perfusion to the brain.

Here's more great news from this study: Our brains are capable of regenerating synapses. Synapses are the microscopic gaps between nerve cells, where electrical impulses pass in the presence of neurotransmitters. Simply put, synapses allow us to remember our schedules, calculate answers to problems, recognize faces, and read a map.

Back in the 1970s, science believed that we all have a finite number of neurons. Once they were gone, whether due to aging, drinking, or whatever, they were gone for good! But recent research has shown that people can grow *new* synapses, and this is more likely in people who practice an active lifestyle.[2]

It almost seems too elementary to think that plain old walking can be so beneficial. The wise father whose mantra was, "Walk it off!" makes me laugh, but I'll be quoting him until I die.

TIPS FOR WALKERS

- A comfortable pair of walking shoes are the only expense for walking, so it's wise to invest in a pair that supports your feet well and feels comfortable. Many sporting goods stores offer expert help with finding the best pair for you.

- Use good posture as you walk. Keep your shoulders back, tummy flat, and feet pointed straight ahead.

- Start your walk with a slow five-minute warm up. When you reach a good pace, you should still be able to carry on a conversation as you walk.

Just Keep Moving!

When it comes to being physically active, let's start where we are and do what we are able to do. Let's not worry that we are not as fast or as fit as our neighbor. We may not walk, swim, or dance with the same grace and ease, but engaging our bodies in physical activity is incredibly important. Plus, it is wonderfully rewarding.

Here are a few facts to nudge us out of our chairs and out the door. In 2010, the best estimate of the global incidence of dementia was 35.6 million people. If these numbers continue to climb as our population ages, that number is predicted to rise to 115.4 million by 2050.[1] It is sobering to think how the weight of the world, literally the weight of our bodies, is stressing society and our health care systems. As more people are living longer, the needs of the elderly population are expanding exponentially. We need to take strides as individuals to do our part to live as healthfully as possible.

No medication can prevent dementia, but research indicates that moving our patooties can. Vascular risk factors, namely hypertension, high cholesterol levels, and high BMI (body mass index), correlate with increased levels of dementia, according to thorough research. It is estimated that half of all dementia cases are related to sedentary lifestyles.[2] Aerobic exercise and strength training, especially when combined with good nutrition, help keep minds and bodies operating more efficiently.

As I have visited many retirement communities with family and friends, it has thrilled my heart to see that the most vibrant, interesting, and engaging folks at these places are the ones who frequent the gym. If you want to meet bright and vivacious residents at any retirement center from Florida to Minneapolis, find your way to the workout room, pool, or dance studio. I guarantee you will discover energetic folks who are full of vim and vigor, both physically and intellectually. How inspiring it is to meet 80- and 90-year-olds who swim, cycle, lift weights, run on treadmills, and take Pilates classes. These are the wise ones who keep me from fearing old age.

I love hearing my brother's tales of cross-country ski competitions where spirited skiers with the best form are well into their eighties. These athletes are skiing 50 kilometers, sometimes in tremendously harsh conditions. Their finish times may be slower, but they are not giving up.

This is my dad all over. While he is not a skier, I remember him as a thirtysomething maverick who liked to run. While jogging is completely normal now, back in the 1960s he was the only guy who ran up and down the streets and alleys of our South Chicago suburb. He had neither proper running shoes nor Lycra clothing. He ran in whatever he happened to wear that day: corduroys or khaki shorts, and usually a collared shirt. Style never crossed his mind; getting his heart pumping did. My mom said the neighbors thought he was crazy. She requested, "Could he please run after dark?" Ha! He simply needed his daily dose of endorphins, and even my mom could not stand in the way of that.

I remember being eight and joining him for his afternoon run one sunny Saturday. As we jogged down an alley, I heard kids call to their friends, "Hey, here comes Jogging Man. Oh, and today he has a Jogging Girl!" Such freaks we were, pounding the pavement and looking ridiculous, but smiling all the way.

In the 1970s, Dad worked in downtown Chicago. He rode the commuter train, which provided the perfect opportunity for daily aerobic exercise. Each morning he hiked a mile to the station. Next he put in another mile from Union Station to his office. His daily four miles on foot gave him energy and plenty of mood elevating endorphins.

In every decade, Dad has continued to keep moving. When aching knees didn't allow for running, he continued to swim, bike, and walk. Several significant rides eventually wore out a knee to the point where he needed a replacement. Even with a new knee joint, however, he kept walking and cycling. When the new joint became infected, it had to be replaced again. This time his leg couldn't bend beyond 90 degrees. At this point, most people would give up. But Dad's drive to keep active, not just for his body but for his mind, spurs him on to walk, swim, lift weights, and ride an indoor bike.

Like many other active seniors, he knows that the antidote to becoming a couch potato is movement. Yes, he misses flying down Elm Street on his bike, and he would dearly love to take one more biking vacation in Europe, but he is doing the best he can with what his body allows. I'm grateful for my aging athlete of a dad, who lives with pain and a body that doesn't cooperate as well as it used to.

He pushes himself physically, which helps him live as healthfully as he can.

May we all follow his example.

Let's Dance

Last year, my husband and I attended a beautiful wedding that was followed by a memorable dinner dance. What made this special was a dance in which each married guest was invited to dance with his or her spouse. As the DJ welcomed couples onto the dance floor, it became a happy, multigenerational crowd swaying to the music, each couple dancing in their own particular way. Next, the DJ invited those who had been married for a day or less to take a seat. Down went the bridal couple, giving them front row seats from which to watch their guests.

As the song continued, with its romantic strains swirling over and around us, we were instructed to depart the dance according to the number of years married. The glamorous ones who had been together only five years or fewer stepped away. Next those married 10 or fewer years…followed by many 40- and 50-year-olds who had 20 years of marriage under their belts.

The number of dancers continued to diminish until, finally, one adorable elderly couple remained on the floor. They didn't twirl the fastest, but their smooth moves spoke of comfort with each other as they anticipated each step. There was no need to fight for the lead. Instead, a peaceful expression lit their faces as they glided around the dance floor, enjoying its entire space. They didn't seem to notice anyone but each other. This drew in their audience all the more. This is the dance that warms my heart more than any other I've seen. It is the one that gives the rest of us hope in a long love that grows with years. It's not flashy, but it is steady and beautiful.

I wondered if this couple danced very often. They certainly seemed to know what they were doing, and they looked like they were having fun. As I watched, it crossed my mind that besides knowing the satisfying joy of moving to the music with one's veteran partner, they were doing what researchers have called the best physical activity of all for the brain and the body.

Because dancing requires repeated rapid-fire decision making, it promotes constant activity along our neural pathways. Synapses fire away over and over as the dance proceeds. Mini decisions are being made in the dancers' brains, promoting stimulation of complex neural pathways. The more complex, the better. Think of it this way: We are trying to cross a creek on a series of stepping-stones. Each stone represents a synaptic connection between our neurons. The more rocks available to us, the greater number of ways we can cross. As we age, some neurons fall into disuse and die (think of rocks being removed). But if there are many rocks, or neural pathways to choose from, we can still make it across.

Similarly, during ballroom dancing, we actively use many neural pathways, keeping neurons alive and well. Lots of functioning pathways equal fewer neurons falling into disuse and sinking into the stream. This is why *The New England Journal of Medicine* published findings from a study done at the Albert Einstein College. This study indicated that aging adults who regularly engage in partner dancing are 76 percent less likely to develop dementia. The cardiac workout and quick neural activity used in dancing is a winning combination.[1]

A unique aspect of ballroom dancing is that it requires one person to lead and one to follow. We might think that only the leader decides which direction the couple will go, but both partners are making quick decisions as they dance. A good leader will be attentive to what works well for his partner, adapting his style to hers. The follower must sense where her partner is leading. It is a give-and-take, symbiotic relationship. Both dancers benefit from the split-second decisions.

Whether a couple is dancing a waltz, salsa, cha-cha, swing, or rhumba, being observant and interpreting a partner's signals provides an excellent mental workout.

In dancing, we can certainly apply the rule, "Use it or lose it." When neural pathways are stimulated, the activity is life-giving on a microscopic level in the brain. The hippocampus, the special seahorse-shaped area of the brain that's associated with memory, and the cerebral cortex, which is responsible for motor movement, intelligence, language, and sensory processing are activated as we dance. This means they rewire themselves according to their use. The more complex the series of decisions, the more complex the pathways that are formed, resulting in a fully functioning brain.[2]

Perhaps dancing has never been your thing. Or if you dance, you fall into ruts of using the same memorized steps every time. Why not try mixing it up? Changing partners is one way to keep you on your toes, literally, as well as sharpen your mind. Varying partners demands greater attention to another person's interpretation of the music. More split-second decisions must be made. This encourages greater neuroplasticity (the ability to form and reorganize our brains' synaptic connections).

Perhaps the best part of dancing is the fun social interaction it provides. Even if you don't have a steady dance partner, there are many places to find others who like to dance. Who knew that minimizing the chances of dementia could be so much fun? So keep dancing. Or *start* dancing.

Green Thumb, Bright Mind

Some of the sharpest people I know are those who love to garden. In fact, they are more than sharp. They are the way-cool people who wear a peaceful expression on their faces and a funny floppy sun-hat on their heads.

There is Ken, a plant-loving botanist, with his myriad dahlias and his vast patch of fragrant raspberries. I know another dahlia expert who lives in Denmark. Her name is Karin-Margareta, and she is my dad's cousin. Her perennial garden looks like the cover of a gardening magazine, with vast bunches of blooms bouncing in the sea breeze that blows constantly on her island.

My friend Bonnie June knows her flowers as though they are dear old friends, which they are. She is a lovely flower herself, giving joyfully to others wherever she goes. One day she appeared on my front porch, holding a planter of "oranges and lemons" blanket flowers. Talk about a pretty sight! And then there are Joan and Jack, who have covered at least an acre with a beautiful bevy of daffodils. In spring their house is surrounded in gold, cream, and bright yellow.

One more gardener shines brightly in my mind's eye: Grandpa Ed. He is a persevering guy who coaxes oodles of potatoes, beets, tomatoes, blackberries, and loads of other produce from the rocky soil in Michigan's Upper Peninsula, where the growing season is as short as a sigh. His potatoes are so delicious they steal center stage from a perfectly grilled steak.

So what do these wonderful workers of the land have in common?

Obviously they love to get outdoors to sink their hands deep in the soil. Something so elemental, so seasonally established as planting seeds and watching them magically sprout green leaves—and develop into plants and eventually produce flowers or food—nourishes the soul on many levels. Being outdoors in nature touches the core of who we are as humans. Feeling the breeze, smelling the earth as it comes to life in the spring, hearing birds and chipmunks, and sensing the loveliness of God's creativity all around us is incredibly therapeutic. For all these aesthetic reasons, gardening is a great stress reliever, but it's more than that. Amazingly enough, when our hands work the soil, our brains receive a dose of serotonin in places that control our mood. This is what antidepressant drugs accomplish—but much more clumsily. Tending roses or raspberries seems a lot more enjoyable than taking pills.

Another reason our friends who garden look so healthy is that gardeners eat more fruits and vegetables than other people do. Yes, they have more fruits and veggies available because of what they grow, but gardeners are just more in touch with what is best to eat. Have you ever heard a gardener talk with vegetable farmers at a farmers' market? Both sides have a lot to say! Enthusiasm bubbles out as they discuss a new variety of peppers, or how the recent rain has caused berries to swell. Such excitement over fresh produce is contagious.

And, of course, the physical aspect of gardening is so good for us. We tote bags of compost around the yard and bend to pull weeds and drop seeds into the soil. Gardening encourages us to be outside and breathe deeply as the physical exercise strengthens us. It beckons us to escape our insular modern existence. When we pull on a pair of tall gumboots and play in dirt, we're like children discovering the beauty of the earth that God made for us to enjoy.

Gardening is good for our bodies. It's good for our souls, and it's certainly good for our minds. Two particular studies followed 60- and 70-year-olds for 16 years. Researchers discovered that those who gardened had a 36 to 74 percent lower risk of having dementia than those who didn't garden, even when other health risks were factored in.[1] In the garden-friendly country of the Netherlands, research points to the stress-lowering effects of working the soil. During one research study, two groups of adults were given a stress-inducing problem to solve. Half of the adults were sent outside to work in a garden. The other half read for pleasure in a quiet place indoors for the same amount of time.

The researchers next compared the anxiety levels of the readers and the gardeners. It was overwhelmingly clear that the gardeners experienced less anxiety than the readers. This anecdotal evidence was confirmed by a simple blood test that showed a decreased level of the stress-producing hormone cortisol in those who worked in the garden. This is why 80 percent of people who garden report they are content with their lives, compared with 6 percent of those who don't garden at all.

A few other benefits of gardening come in such tiny packages that they are invisible. When we are outdoors, we take in microscopic goodies—gifts from nature that we don't see. When the sun shines on us, our skin magically manufactures the all-important vitamin D, which is really a hormone. This critical vitamin does myriad wonders for our bodies. It promotes bone health, strengthens our immunity, helps fight cancer, and encourages us to feel more positive. It seems fair to call a vitamin D supplement a "happy pill," though it is even more heroic than that.

Additionally, gardeners come into contact with a friendly microbe called Mycobacterium vaccae. It is harmless bacteria found in soil. When we touch it or inhale it as we work the earth, it produces serotonin, the chemical that soothes our minds and keeps our mood on an even keel.[2]

A study in Norway allowed a group of people who had been diagnosed with depression to garden for six hours a week for three months. Half of the group experienced considerable relief from depression. When retested three months later, these folks were still feeling good.[3]

I don't think any of us needs to feel particularly blue to see that gardening is good for our entire being. No matter what season we are in, growing plants in soil is a wonderful thing to do. If it's warm today, get outside and into the dirt! If it is the dead of winter, treat your mind and soul to a pot of herbs, a countertop terrarium, or a little Norfolk pine that will bring the outdoors in. If you live in a city that has a conservatory or greenhouse, stroll through its tropical environment to calm your heart and encourage your spirit until the springtime thaw, when you can pull on your boots and go outdoors.

Pilates...Yes, Please!

It's my guess that you have either taken a Pilates class and loved it, or you wonder what in the world it is. Some years ago, I wandered into a Pilates studio at the recommendation of a cycle-spinning and running coach. He described it as "ballet for athletes." That day I discovered a form of exercise that has been part of my morning routine ever since. It serves me well in mind, body, and spirit. It wakes me up. It stretches and strengthens my muscles and prepares me mentally for the day ahead. And it makes me a little less klutzy.

This is how Pilates began: In 1883, Joseph Pilates was born in Germany. By his own admission, he was born about 50 years ahead of his time. As a boy, he suffered miserably with asthma, but he pushed himself athletically, desiring to grow healthy and strong. By the time he reached adulthood, he was an avid skier, gymnast, diver, and boxer. As he grew athletically and studied many types of exercise, Joseph became fascinated by the Greek philosophy that a healthy person is balanced in mind, body, and spirit. He strived to develop exercises that would strengthen those three facets. He developed unique exercise classes that were well received by the elite dance community in Germany. When he immigrated to the US in the early 1920s, he opened an exercise studio in New York City. Once again, leading dancers and athletes rushed to his door. The popularity of Pilates, which Joe originally called "Contrology," continued to grow. Eventually it became the rage in Los Angeles as well as New York.[1]

Dancers such as Martha Graham and George Balanchine, as well as many professional athletes, realized that Joe Pilates's exercises helped heal sore muscles and prevent injuries. They also found that Pilates calms the mind and decreases stress. Pilates draws on the concept of engaging our brains as we exercise, particularly focusing on our core: the abdominal muscles and muscles around the spine. Pilates dubbed these muscles the "power house." This includes all the muscles from the shoulders down to the glutes. When our core is strong, it is easy to stand tall with excellent posture. Extending from the power house are the arms and legs, which are toned to be long and lean, rather than thick and bulky like a weight-lifter's muscles. Pilates targets almost every muscle group. Even the feet and ankles get a workout.

As we stretch and strengthen muscles the Pilates way, we also engage the brain. This encourages a positive balance between the mind and body—and I would add *spirit*.

The six principles of Pilates are: centering (mentally focusing on the core muscles), concentration, control, precision, breath, and flow. The way we extend our legs or hold our abdominal muscles tight is much more important than number of repetitions. Quality beats quantity. Also, the slow, sustained movements, often carried out on a mat on the floor, are beautiful and gentle, never jerking muscles and causing pain or injury. As we work various muscle groups, we breathe slowly and deeply, releasing anxiety and stress as we focus on the strength that moves from the center of us, outward. Sometimes we must concentrate to tighten one muscle while releasing another. This keeps our minds in the game.[2]

As we lean into these exercises, our brains benefit from a nice surge of endorphins. Also, tension in shoulders, neck, back, and hips decrease as our mind focuses on the flow of movements. The mental rewards are real. Pilates draws the mind and body into a balanced awareness of one another.

For example, we commonly hold tension in our neck, back, and hips. This begins innocently as we attempt to remain socially confident and in control of our world. Let's say you are a teacher, and your group of children turns wildly rambunctious just as the school principal steps into your classroom. Suddenly, "fight-or-flight" hormones flood your system. You know that neither fight nor flight is a good option, so (subconsciously) your breathing becomes shallow. Your shoulders rise and tense up, and your lower back and hips tighten. You may not deeply exhale until the school day has ended and you're driving home. That's when a lower backache makes its presence known. You say, "Where did *that* come from?" It came from holding tension, which your body would be glad to release.

A great way to free ourselves of tension is proper breathing. Joe Pilates felt that breathing deeply and rhythmically while exercising is paramount. He was known to say, "If you do anything right, let it be breathing." He was sure that most of us go through life inhaling and exhaling according to the stress we feel at any given moment. We need to let it go!

I hope I haven't made Pilates sound difficult to do, because it's not. For me it's the most enjoyable way to start the day. No matter where I am, I spread out a fleece blanket, turn on some relaxing music and start in, extending my legs, pointing my toes, tightening "power house," and relaxing the muscles in my shoulders. I move through a routine that has become as natural as breathing.

For me, the best aspect of Pilates is its influence on the way I stand, sit, walk, and think. It makes me comfortable in my own skin. It's similar to a self-fulfilling prophecy. It's easier to stand up straight because my core is supporting me well. And, because I can stand tall, I feel better. I have more confidence and a greater sense of peace in my soul. My husband hears me stumble out of bed and do my Pilates, and only then am I able to walk correctly.

A PILATES PRIMER

- It's worth it to take a few classes to learn correct Pilates techniques.

- Pilates can be modified for any level of flexibility or athletic ability.

- It is easy to do Pilates anywhere (even in hotel rooms, at the beach, or in the backyard).

- Attend a Pilates class with a friend. Enjoy a fruit smoothie afterward.

- If you prefer not to go to a Pilates studio or gym, find a class on YouTube.

- You can probably check out a Pilates DVD from your local library.

Nap-Time Miracles

How ironic it is that preschoolers vehemently resist nap time, while adults would dearly love to lie down and zone out for one blessed and cozy half hour. I imagine we all remember being a small child and getting tucked into bed on a sunny summer afternoon, knowing we were missing something extraordinarily fun. At least that's how it was for me. I could hear my big sister and brother splashing in the blow-up pool outside my bedroom window without me. Nap time felt like unfair punishment for being born third.

Fast-forward 16 years to living in a college dorm, keeping college-student hours. Naps were survival! Between classes I would jog back to my dorm room, lie down on my bed, and breathe deeply a few times to lower my heart rate. In a moment, a pleasant cloud of dreams surrounded me, lifting my mind out of the present for five blissful minutes. While my little power naps were shorter than what most people need, my alarm awoke me just in time to run to my next class, feeling wonderfully refreshed and able to fully engage in the lecture and discussion. If I skipped my five-minute repose, I struggled hard to focus in class. My head bobbed as my body leaned into nap mode right there in front of my professor and classmates.

It is a known fact that a 15- to 20-minute nap does wonders for the human brain. Research has proven that energy, alertness, and productivity (which tend to slump after lunchtime) are easily restored by a short nap. Especially in our sleep-deprived society, we are prone to fatigue and drowsiness in the middle of the day. After a nap, however, we return to our tasks with sharper minds and increased creativity and ability to learn. Research proves that a nap even decreases anxiety by minimizing levels of cortisol, that "stress hormone" that increases blood sugar levels.[1]

Many high-profile and highly successful individuals are sworn nappers. Winston Churchill, Thomas Edison, Yogi Berra, and Margaret Thatcher all accomplished more because of daily naps. More and more companies have followed their example and provide nap rooms in the workplace. They report greater productivity, with fewer employees nodding off at their computers or in a meeting.

In the offices of Google, well-designed sleep pods provide quiet places for workers to stretch out without having to leave the campus. Google believes the middle-of-the-day siesta helps keep people's brains in the game, especially during the last few hours of the workday. An architectural firm in Kansas City has "spent tents" complete with pillows and blankets for comfortable, easy-access naps in a quiet area of their offices. They, too, find that employees who grab a few winks after lunch work more efficiently.

That said, it's worth mentioning that effective midday shut-eye requires a bit of strategy. Not all catnaps do the trick. In fact, some people are sworn non-nappers because at some point they napped too late in the day, and it ruined their nighttime sleep. And all of us, at one time or another, have overindulged in an extended nap and woke feeling groggy and worse than when we dozed off.

We need to be nap savvy and understand what is happening in our brains when we take a midday slide into the land of nod.

For one thing, our sleep is arranged in an undulating pattern. On a graph, it looks like a row of steep mountain peaks. Each peak represents about 90 minutes. The deep valleys between the peaks are when we are in deep sleep, unconscious to the world. None of us does well when we are jolted out of this deep valley of slumber. Rather, if we can time our naps so we wake up during light sleep, depicted by the mountain peaks, we feel refreshed and ready to resume activities with a clear head. So a 90-minute midday nap is particularly beneficial when we are learning new material. While napping, the brain miraculously takes newly learned ideas and concepts from our short-term memory bank in the hippocampus, sorts through them, and files them neatly in our long-term memory storage area in the brain's cortex.[2] It's amazing! This process frees up space in "short-term parking" for new material to be taken in.

Research has also proven that good sleep before learning clears the clutter in our short-term memory bank, preparing it to absorb fresh information.

Both kinds of naps were my friends during intense periods of absorbing information as a nursing student. The 5- to 15-minute power naps between classes increased my mental alertness. My strategy for mastering long lists of nerves, bones, muscles, and medications went like this: First, I wrote them on flash cards, which my husband quizzed me on before we went to sleep. Next, I tucked them under my pillow to let osmosis do the rest. I "slept on it," literally.

While my mind dreamed of dancing wildly on a remote beach far from school, my brain took those crazy flash card words and stuck them neatly in the cortex of my brain. Those facts were settled nicely into place by the next morning, when I needed them for a test or in a clinical at the hospital. This concept still thrills me!

So let's do our brains a favor and avoid fighting naps as though we're preschoolers afraid of missing a good time. Feel free to grab a fleece blanket and wrap yourself up for 20 minutes of much-needed rest. The energy gained by a few midday Z's will be worth the minutes you borrow from your daily schedule.

SLEEP ON THIS!

- Some of us take a longer time to fall asleep than others. If you need 10 minutes to get to sleep, add that time to your 15-minute nap.
- If you are sleep deprived, a short nap is more effective than drinking coffee or an energy drink.
- The benefits of a 15-minute catnap include greater alertness for up to four hours.

"You Smoke like Smelly the Bear!"

One night, after sitting by a campfire, my husband, Eric, and I were putting our little boys to bed. Three-year-old Bjorn stuck his nose into my hair and said, "Mommy, you smoke like Smelly the Bear!" Between gales of laughter over his innocent twisting of words, we tried to explain that it's "Smokey the Bear" whose fragrance I wore. And yes, it was smelly. That's when we started the no-smoking campaign with our children. Through the years, we pointed out the commonly known facts that smoking is bad for our lungs, and it causes heart disease. It increases the chance of having many kinds of cancer. It ruins the voice, prematurely ages the skin, and is highly addictive. But what we missed conveying to our kids, simply because we were unaware, is that smoking damages the brain.

Smoking is detrimental to brain health in a variety of ways. When a person smokes, it takes about 10 seconds for 600 chemicals in each cigarette to reach the brain. One hundred of these chemicals have a negative pharmacological effect on the brain, an effect that is evident for days. Carbon monoxide in cigarette smoke binds with red blood cells, so oxygen cannot. This robs the brain of oxygen and causes a buildup of carbon dioxide. Nicotine also stimulates the central nervous system by interfering with neurotransmitters. This releases dopamine and endorphins, making a smoker feel *momentarily* mellow. But the brain gets used to this fleeting bliss, and soon a person must smoke more to feel normal. Nicotine is as addictive as heroin.

In addition to these microscopic effects, smoking thins the brain's cerebral cortex, a 2- to 4-millimeter covering between the brain and the skull. We recognize the cerebral cortex by its folds and creases. This cortex is responsible for key thinking skills, including problem solving, voluntary movement, language, attention, and memory. We know that the cerebral cortex becomes thinner as a person ages, but smoking accelerates this process. Also, a study at the University of Edinburgh, Scotland, which involved 250 smokers and 250 nonsmokers, found a strong correlation between smoking and brain decline—leading to dementia and even Alzheimer's disease. The study also revealed that those who stopped smoking, even in their seventies, were able to begin *immediate* healing of the brain. For light smokers, it took only a matter of weeks for the brain to recover. But for those who smoked a pack a day, it took up to 25 years to reverse smoking's evil effects on the brain.

This good news about the positive results of smoking cessation encourages anyone to stop smoking, but especially those in middle age, who still have time to restore the health of their brains.

Unfortunately, because nicotine is so addictive, quitting is difficult. Moreover, smokers fear weight gain if they give it up. It's true that smoking increases metabolism and decreases appetite. But weight gain associated with quitting is only seven to ten pounds. People who have successfully kicked the habit encourage others to work on quitting first and *then* think about weight loss. In other words, one thing at a time. Start with what is most detrimental to your health.[1]

As I grew up, no one in my family smoked, so the smell of cigarettes holds few but surprisingly nice memories. For many years, my parents and six of their best friends had a dinner club that rotated from one home to the next. Two of the men smoked, so my mom brought out a couple of beautiful ashtrays whenever she hosted. The fragrance of standing rib roast mingled with wisps of cigarette smoke floated up to the kids' bedrooms, where my siblings and I, freshly scrubbed, played board games on our beds. Remembering the happy chatter and the heavenly food smells and cigarettes seems pleasantly nostalgic. While smoking in restaurants has all but disappeared in the United States, a trip to Europe last summer brought back that nostalgic mix of aromas from my childhood.

But here is the stark reality: As my parents and their friends grew older, members of their dinner club began to die. It wasn't a shock when the first to go was the man who had been the heaviest smoker. He was followed by his wife, who breathed a lot of secondhand smoke. The next to die was the other gentleman who smoked, though not as much. His daughter and I are lifelong friends, and once, to send her dad a "no smoking" message, we swiped a pack of his cigarettes. We unwrapped it, cut each cigarette in half, soaked them in water, and returned them to the pack. But it takes more than two mischievous sixth graders to effect change.

No doubt, smoking shortens lives, but it also diminishes quality of life as it poisons the brain. Even if you don't quit for yourself, know that your family will be grateful that you don't "smoke like Smelly the bear."

IF YOU NEED TO QUIT SMOKING...

- Check with your physician or local hospital about ways to quit.
- Don't try to do it alone. Seek the support of a group.
- Remember that many smoking-induced damages to the brain are reversible.

Breathe

Breathing exercises were such a great help when I delivered my first baby that soon afterward I became a childbirth instructor at our local hospital. It was one of the most rewarding jobs ever. During six weekly sessions, it was my privilege to help expectant parents prepare for the birth of their babies by sharing knowledge and techniques to support them through labor and birth. We discussed maternal physiology and what to expect during the remainder of the pregnancy. But mostly we practiced special ways of breathing. The breathing techniques included inhaling slowly through the nose and out through the mouth. We practiced short, staccato breathing for the height of painful contractions, and we practiced long, sustained exhalations for delivery. I encouraged the moms in my weekly pumpkin patch to practice their breathing so it would become second nature when the moment of need arrived.

Simply *breathing*—you may wonder how that could possibly make a difference in the pain of childbirth. It certainly did for me. The breathing exercises and my husband's presence by my side got me through three times. But as soon as the baby enters the world, what is our most elemental concern? Ironically, everyone in the birthing room holds their breath waiting for the infant to take its first breath. Finally, when the baby breathes, so do the rest of us, gasping with great relief! To breathe is to live. To breathe deeply from the bottom of the diaphragm is to live well and to promote brain health at the same time.

Breathing is something we do all the time, so it may seem superfluous to discuss this most basic human need. But the way we inhale and exhale has great impact on our health. Have you ever considered that breathing is voluntary and involuntary? We breath without thinking about it…or we can alter our breathing by doing it fast, slow, shallow, or deep. We might even hold our breath, but if we hold it for too long, we'll pass out and our body will unconsciously resume breathing for us. (I think God built in this safety feature for middle schoolers who attempt to impress each other with such antics.)

Let's consider the voluntary aspect of breathing—the part we can control. A good deep breath from the depths of the diaphragm gives the body a full dose of oxygen and gets rid of carbon dioxide. At the doctor's office, the glowing clip placed on your finger measures the amount of oxygen in your blood. If you want to get a great reading, take a nice long deep breath, in through the nose to the count of five, hold it for a moment, and exhale slowly through the mouth, taking a bit longer on the exhalation than on the inhalation. As you do this, more oxygen enters the body and more carbon dioxide exits. This kind of deep breathing does our bodies a lot of good.

First of all, it helps relieve stress. We are controlled by both the sympathetic and the parasympathetic nervous systems. The sympathetic, or fight-or-flight response, stands by at all times, prepared to be deployed should an alarming situation arise. On the flip, our parasympathetic system has a calming effect, keeping us from freaking out unnecessarily. If we live too much in fight-or-flight mode, the cortisol or stress hormone level in the brain is elevated, which can impair memory, decrease our ability to problem solve, wreck our mood, and promote weight gain and insomnia. Being constantly stressed can even lead to depression.

Research proves however, that relaxation breathing engages the parasympathetic nervous system by stimulating the vagal nerve, which runs from the brain to the abdomen. This nerve releases acetylcholine, which promotes greater mental focus and a calming effect on our minds and bodies. When we are calm, we are less likely to entertain anxious thoughts. As a result, our blood pressure and heart rate decrease, giving our circulatory system a healthy break. This in turn lowers the risk of stroke.

Also, regular deep breathing promotes thickening of the gray matter of the brain, similar to when musicians play their music and jugglers juggle. The extra oxygen to the brain sparks neural growth, which leads to more effective brain function. A research study at the Feinberg School of Medicine at Northwestern University in Chicago discovered a significant difference between brain activity during inhalation and exhalation.[1] As we breathe in, the neurons in the olfactory cortex (the area of the brain that tells us we smell something before we can identify it), the amygdala (which influences memory, decision making, and emotional reactions), and the hippocampus (the all-important memory center) are stimulated. If you are straining to remember something that has slipped your mind, try taking a few sustained breaths in through your nose and exhale slowly through your mouth. During the inhalation part of breathing, a greater concentration of oxygen reaches your brain, and you have a better chance of recalling the missing thought.

Improving memory and decreasing stress and anxiety simply by adopting a few simple breathing exercises seems like a no-brainer to me. Actually not a no-brainer...more like a "yes-brainer."

When you find yourself in a stressful moment, no matter what the cause, train yourself to stop and breathe deeply. Inhale slowly through your nose as you silently count to five. Hold the breath for a moment before exhaling slowly through your mouth. As you exhale, allow your shoulders to relax. Think about places in your body where you hold tension, and let it go. Repeat five to ten times as you are able. Include deep breathing exercises in your morning routine to start the day in peace. Since my husband began doing this a year ago, he has even developed better breath support for singing and public speaking.

More Than a Helmet

Your ability to read this book proves that you're a giant step ahead of the much-beloved scarecrow from Oz who says (and sings), "If I only had a brain." Ironically, for not having a brain, he is quite aware of all he'd like to think and do. His insight about the complex gift of a brain reminds us how important it is to be able to think. But I wonder if we consider the many ways we need to take good care of our brains.

For me, growing up on a bicycle meant glorious freedom. I can still see the bike of my youth and Elm Street Hill, which brought me home, lickety-split. I went down that hill as fast as I could, no hands on the handlebars, invincible and fearless. I still like to bike after dark through woods and over bridges. It's the joy of youth extended. One difference, however, is the addition of a helmet closely fit to my head, strap snug under my chin. It's 12 ounces of brain protection absolutely required at our house.

Not too long ago, the value of the bike helmet was hammered home when we were cycling with our two twentysomething boys. I put an apple pie in the oven, and we took off for a 45-minute ride while it baked. On the way home, I yelled ahead to the guys, "Apple pie!" They took off like a shot. Within a half mile I regretted my announcement, as my husband and I came upon the terrifying sight of one son bent over the other, who was sprawled between trees on the side of the bike trail. Blood gushed from his face. He didn't know who we were.

I rubbed his hands and felt his head, grateful he was breathing, as we waited for the ambulance. It was a long night in the trauma center as Karl-Jon endured sutures to his face, X-rays, and CAT scans. When, at two in the morning, he started singing a ridiculous song, I knew his sense of humor was returning and that the cuts and broken bones around his eye would heal. When the doctor asked what happened, Karl-Jon replied in all honesty, "I have a propensity to let my mind wander." The doc gave me a quizzical sideways grin, and remarked, "Uh-huh. Klutzy, and maybe a little spacy, but intelligent!"

That night and at every follow-up visit, Karl-Jon was asked the same question: "Were you wearing a helmet?" When the maxillofacial surgeon heard the affirmative "Yes," he looked Karl-Jon square in his injured face and said, "I believe it saved your life!" Wow. I shudder to think. And I wonder at everyone's survival of childhood.

We can protect our brains on many levels, from physical to biochemical. Much of this book covers the importance of brain preservation on the cellular level. Eating healthfully to keep cholesterol, blood sugar levels, and weight under control *matters*. So does limiting alcohol consumption and never smoking. Outdoor exercise, getting our heart rate up, deep breathing, and staying connected with others also count. But so does protecting the actual melon that sits on top of our shoulders.

As our boys learned firsthand, wearing a helmet is important. It should always be part of playing contact sports. And it shouldn't be neglected when we cycle, skateboard, snowboard, snowmobile, and ride a horse or any vehicle, such as an ATV or a motorcycle. Multiple concussions sustained when young can negatively influence brain health later in life. Increased concern for football and hockey players who routinely take blows to the head has been making headlines. Several studies indicate that athletes who suffer head injuries may be at greater risk for mild cognitive impairment, which often leads to dementia.[1]

As our ski buddy Lee says, "Do you have a $25 head or a $250 head? Get a decent helmet!"

For folks over 65, two-thirds of hospitalizations in the state of New

York are related to falls, most of which happen in the home.[2] When reaching for a top shelf, use a solid step stool. As we get older, our balance is not what it used to be. Learning a few simple exercises to improve balance is an easy way to prevent a fall. Also, throw rugs, loose handrails, or the absence of handrails can be hazardous. It's important to take a good look around your living environment to note anything that could cause a fall. Good lighting helps, especially around stairways, which should be kept clear. Check for a cords, rumpled rugs, and uneven carpeting. And as much as pets offer unconditional love and companionship, especially for those who might live alone, we need to take extra care to avoid tripping over a dog or a cat.

Even Queen Elizabeth II, who has been inseparable from her devoted corgis and dorgis, is down to three dogs, and she is not replacing them once they are gone.

If you live in a place where the temperature gets below freezing, it's a good idea to keep a bucket of sand and salt ready to sprinkle on outdoor stairs and walkways. Slipping and falling on ice is the number one cause of brain injury in northern states, and it happens to people of all ages.[3]

As I continue to bike the trail where our son wiped out, I never see the tree he narrowly missed without thanking God for the helmet that may have saved his life. The helmet was a lot easier to replace than Karl-Jon's precious head.

Sleep Matters

Sometimes getting enough shut-eye seems like a losing battle. As we pack our days full, attempting to complete all our tasks, we often sacrifice sleep. But research is beginning to reveal amazing neurochemical activity that takes place in our brains *only* while we sleep. In very simple terms, sleep is when the neurological trash in our brains is taken out.[1]

Our brain has two operating modes: It's awake and alert, or it's asleep and cleaning up. It's like my local post office: It's either open for business or locked up for the night. There is no middle ground. If I come to mail a package two minutes after the door is locked, I am out of luck.

As I peer in the post-office window at this unfortunate hour, I'll see bins of letters and packages stacked up and waiting to go. The post office is closed, but the postal workers are still working. They scurry to sort and truck our mail across town or to the airport, directing each piece to its destination. I still find the postal service to be a miracle of our modern world. And Amazon? Don't get me started! But one thing is for sure: If I'm the first customer to mail my box the next morning, all the counters and conveyers will be clear of mail. All the bins will be empty. It's a fresh start each morning as my post office opens for business.

Similarly, each day our brains take in thousands of stimuli—visual and auditory, what we taste, what we feel, and what we are challenged to think about. There is so much input that the brain cannot process the tsunami of thoughts and feelings as fast as they arrive. But even more amazing is what happens to the enormous variety of details when we sleep. As soon as the sandman ushers us into the land of nod, our brains get busy sorting and cataloging the information they received that day. A lot happens while one's head is on the pillow. In fact, parts of our brains are busier while we are asleep than when we're awake. Memories are stored, problems are solved, insights are gained, and attention is given to details.

The process by which this happens has eluded scientists for years. But with the use of two-photon microscopy, scientists have discovered the unique plumbing, or glymphatic system, by which the brain is cleared of the potentially neurotoxic waste that accumulates while we are awake. When we sleep, whether naturally or while under anesthesia, the cells in the brain shrink to give cerebrospinal fluid ample room to flow freely between cells and remove the crud. It's like getting our cars off the street during a snowstorm to make room for the plow to come in and clean up.

This "brain snow," however, is a protein called amyloid-beta, which, when allowed to pile up, is associated with Alzheimer's disease. In fact, nearly every neurodegenerative disease is associated with an accumulation of cellular waste products.[2]

Much research continues as scientists strive to understand this intricate waste-removal system in our sleeping brains. Mysteries are still being solved. But one thing is certain: Chemical secretions that repair our bodies and brains are imperative for our survival. If we are extremely sleep deprived, the mind and body are likely to spontaneously shut down with disastrous results. This is the body's way of screaming for what it needs. And it needs "brain trash" removal. That's why people who are terribly sleep deprived are at risk for falling asleep while driving. They are also prone to make bad decisions and lose their ability to problem solve. They are trying to function with a "dirty brain."

I've done my fair share of dirty brain survival. It's not fun. High demands during certain seasons of our lives make it tough to get the recommended seven to nine hours of sleep each night. I particularly remember working as a night nurse while starting a family. Interrupted and irregular sleep makes it difficult for young parents to give their brains time to reboot. But as we begin to understand how imperative sleep is for the health of our brains, making it a priority seems more worthwhile. Considering the important neurologic cleanup that takes place during sleep, it's no wonder that if we were sad or stressed at bedtime, my grandma would always say, "Just sleep now. Everything will seem better in the morning." She was right. And if you feel pressured to make a decision before you are ready, you know why answering, "I'll need to sleep on that," is a wise and valid response.

Massage: A Treat for Mind and Body

If I happen to look uncharacteristically blue or needy and my husband asks what I need, my standard answer is, "Eggs Benedict and a good massage!" He assumes I'm joking, and of course I am, but both remedies go a long way to a lift a girl's spirits. While a massage may seem like an unnecessary luxury, the benefits for mind and body are substantial. This is why massage continues to attract the attention of the medical community. Lots of good happens in the body and the brain during a massage. Let me explain.

Therapeutic massage, which is sustained deep rubbing and kneading of the skin and muscle groups, is known to decrease anxiety and help relieve strained or injured muscles. It is often the best way to soothe back pain, and what it does for our brains is highly desirable too. As you probably know, cortisol and adrenaline are stress hormones that jump to action when we feel threatened or stressed. They drop into our blood stream, gifts from our adrenal glands at those "day late, dollar short" moments. Or when the neighbor's mastiff jumps at the fence and threatens to eat you for dinner.

Adrenaline produces a zippy heart rate and increased respiration. Cortisol binds with fat receptors in the liver and the pancreas, releasing glucose to fuel our muscles for a quick getaway. Together these hormones supply the fight-or-flight response that may well save our necks. So during menacing moments, bring them on. But at other times these powerful stress chemicals don't do us any favors. Plenty of people suffer with stress and anxiety and the resulting elevated levels of cortisol. I am not suggesting that a massage is the cure-all for every anxiety, but it certainly helps decrease cortisol levels and knock down stress.[1]

While a massage keeps cortisol in check, it increases the "feel good" neurotransmitters serotonin and dopamine in our brain. Serotonin, which helps us feel peaceful and encourages sleep, also promotes feelings of contentment and well-being. Dopamine rallies around our mental reward system, giving us pleasure and alertness. It is the neurohormone that comes into play as you paint a picture. It sparks inspiration and intuition. Another hormone, oxytocin, which is extra prevalent in pregnant, birthing, and nursing mothers, also abounds during a massage. Oxytocin, sometimes referred to as "the love hormone," promotes feelings of comfort. It encourages us to bond with a new baby or a lover. You can understand why, with the combination of serotonin, dopamine, and oxytocin, we often feel mellowed to a puddle following a massage.

One exception is the 15-minute chair massage, which energizes us with a jump in adrenaline.[2] But a slower, longer, deep-muscle massage drains our adrenaline and may relax us to the point of sleep. Those who fall asleep during a massage exhibit the characteristic delta waves linked with deep sleep. Even during a vigorous, muscle-manipulating massage, this effect is possible thanks to a rise in serotonin.[3]

Science aside, a massage is a wonderful way to relieve stress and soothe aching muscles. If you have never enjoyed a massage, check with your physician for a recommendation.

Before the massage, the therapist will ask you about any tight or painful muscle groups that need particular attention. Also, if you have any injuries or recent surgeries, the therapist will take these into consideration. Most massage studios play soft music and offer aromatherapy. Oil or lotion will be applied to the skin to decrease friction, and it's good to drink a lot of water afterward to flush toxins released by the massage. Eggs Benedict or not, a massage is a treat for the mind and the body. It calms aching muscles and anxious minds.

A MASSAGE PRIMER

- **Swedish:** Gentle, longer strokes, kneading, deeper motions.

- **Deep-tissue massage:** Slower, more forceful strokes. It targets deeper muscle layers and connective tissue.

- **Trigger point massage:** Focuses on knots or tight areas of muscles, resulting from strain or injury.

- **Sport massage:** Similar to Swedish massage, but it focuses on preventing or treating injuries.[4]

Note: A reputable massage therapist should be certified through the National Certification Board for Therapeutic Massage or by the American Massage Therapy Association.[5]

Part Two

Nutrition

Popeye and Mom

Once again, as we contemplate what's best for the brain, we need to consider what's powering the machine. As we aim to eat healthfully, let's picture a dinner plate. A good way to start is to mentally divide the plate in half. Next, cut one of the halves in half, making three sections. One half of the plate is for our vegetables and fruits, with the greatest proportion being veggies. One quarter of the plate holds whole grains, such as whole-wheat pasta, hulled barley, wheat berries, or brown rice. The final quarter is for protein: Fish, poultry, beans, nuts, or, very rarely, red meat. Filling our plate according to this general guideline helps us plan meals that are high in nutrients.[1] Obviously, some foods are better for us than others. In fact, some are so good they've been dubbed "superfoods." Superfoods are calorie sparse and nutrient dense. They are high in antioxidants, vitamins, and minerals. They are super for us because they give us a good bang for our buck nutritionally. And they are readily available at a local grocery store or farmers' market.

Consider the humble egg. Eggs are nature's perfect package of protein. After eating an egg with something whole grain for breakfast, we are more apt to feel full at least until lunchtime. Plus, eggs contain 12 vitamins and minerals, especially choline, which is good for brain development and memory. Other big nutritional hitters are nuts, kiwi, yogurt, quinoa, beans, salmon, broccoli, spinach, kale, sweet potatoes, and berries.

Let's take a closer look at spinach. Popeye threw down whole cans to make his muscles pop. As a kid, I thought my mom was in cahoots with Popeye, dreaming up ways to make spinach more desirable for children. Most of us didn't realize that spinach is not only delicious, it is mighty good for us. A one-cup serving of spinach contains only 41 calories, yet it delivers twice as much iron as other greens. It is also an excellent source of vitamin K, which we need to clot blood. It's packed full of beta-carotene, vitamin C, and folic acid. Some other greens are tasty sources of water, but spinach also delivers manganese, magnesium, and vitamin B2. No wonder so much folklore surrounds spinach and its goodness. From a sixteenth-century Florentine lady who went off to marry the king of France with spinach seeds in her trousseau, to Popeye with his whole-can habit, spinach has a long and solid reputation. It is famous for its ability to increase strength, promote vitality, and improve the quality of our blood. When you see the word "Florentine" on a menu, know that spinach is involved, and so is good nutrition.

Another fabulous green is kale. To place kale in its proper family tree, note that it's actually a smooth-leaved fraternal twin of collard greens and a great-grandchild of wild cabbage, in the cruciferous cabbage family. But its popularity is not based merely on family connections. Kale's unprecedented levels of important nutrients make it a high and mighty champ among its green neighbors in the produce department. Steamed kale is strongly antioxidant. It helps prevent inflammation in the body. These two characteristics have an anti-cancer effect. Kale is also high in calcium and vitamins A, C, B1, B2, and E. Just one cup of kale packs 70 percent of our daily requirement of cold-fighting vitamin C, while it costs the eater a modest 20 calories. Plus, it's high in dietary fiber, which promotes good digestive, cardiac, and brain function.

A wide variety of kale is showing up at farmers' markets these days, so talk to the growers, who are usually experts in what they are selling. If they aren't, move along until you find one who is. Most likely, they grow a particular kind of kale because they like it, and they probably know how to cook it as well. Red Russian kale has reddish purple stems with intricate green leaves. It is most tender and sweet after a frost and needs to be thoroughly cooked to be pleasantly chewy. It's best to steam kale before sautéing it, being sure the kale is cut into pieces that are no larger than a half-inch for the leaves and a quarter-inch for the stems.

This ensures even cooking and doesn't ruin the nutritional value of the kale. Tuscan or Lacinato kale, like most other greens, responds better to gentler cooking. A simple way to prepare it is to braise the chopped kale in a sauté pan with a tiny amount of water and apple slices until the kale is tender. Before serving, drizzle with balsamic vinegar and sprinkle with chopped walnuts. This would make a healthful and tasty dish to accompany a grilled or sautéed chicken breast.

The sky is the limit when it comes to incorporating healthful greens like spinach or kale into our diets. Whether we eat them fresh in cold salads, wilted with olive oil and garlic, or as a bed under fish, these greens are generous providers of the good nutrients our bodies need. And the crazy thing we've discovered at our house is that when we fill up on nutritious meals first, we don't have room in our bellies for the fluffy foods we used to crave.

STRAWBERRY SPINACH SALAD WITH HONEY-LIME VINAIGRETTE DRESSING

Salad

8 oz. baby spinach leaves
1 pint fresh ripe strawberries, cleaned, hulled, and quartered
3 scallions (white and light green parts) cut into thin crosswise slices
½ cup sliced almonds

Toss spinach leaves, strawberry halves, and scallions in a large salad bowl. Reserve almonds.

Honey-Lime Vinaigrette Dressing

juice and zest of one lime
3 T. canola oil
3 T. honey
pinch of salt

Place vinaigrette ingredients into a jar. Shake to combine. Just before serving, dress the salad and sprinkle almonds over the top.

Serves 6.

Woes of the Western Diet

W hat's on the menu, darling?"

"The Western diet? Yikes, I'm out of here!"

That ought to be our response, but that's rarely the case. Most of us don't know what the so-called Western diet is, so how can we understand why it's a poor choice for maintaining a healthy body and a sound mind?

Generally speaking, this diet has been encroaching on us since the end of World War II, when our food production became much more automated and driven by big business. No longer was it easy for subsistence farms or small family farms to survive. Our food started to come by way of enormous corporations touting convenience cooking over quality or nutritional value.

Today, not many of us question the origins of our food. Instead we are accustomed to giant supermarkets with entire aisles dedicated to machine-extruded cereals that have no resemblance to the grains from which they came. Of course, procuring food for our families is more convenient than it was in 1930, but are we eating as healthfully? Sadly, we are not.

As the medical community bends under the strain of enormous increases in the incidence of obesity and Alzheimer's disease, researchers are working hard to discover where we have gone off the rails nutritionally. With over one-third of our American adult population now tipping the scales into the obese range, researchers are scrambling to understand this epidemic. Along with obesity comes all kinds of metabolic issues, including glucose intolerance and insulin resistance, which often precede diabetes. High triglycerides and cholesterol levels are out of control. So is hypertension. But the bad news does not stop here. Alzheimer's disease, which now affects more than 5 million Americans, is likely to increase fourfold in the next 40 years. The price tag for us as individuals, as a nation, and globally is astronomical.[1]

In daily conversations, I hear many thoughtful folks comment that the incidence of Alzheimer's is off the charts and we don't understand why. Actually, medical research is uncovering truth about what we eat and how it directly influences the way our minds and bodies work. When we follow the rapid global shift from diets high in fiber and complex carbohydrates (fruits, veggies, and whole grains) to diets that have proportionally more fats and refined sugars (burgers and fries), we not only alter our waistlines but also wreak havoc on our brains.[2]

Don't get me wrong. I love a warm chocolate chip cookie as much as anyone, but we all need to take a good honest look at what we're consuming if we want to preserve our cognitive abilities. Research is pointing to diet's long-term influence on the brain. First, when we eat foods full of sugar and saturated fat, the brain's self-regulating glucose system goes haywire. Without it, the brain doesn't tell us, "Stop eating!"

Also, the number of cells that help neurons grow and thrive are depleted. Neuroinflammation, which is associated with Alzheimer's, sets in. This inflammation causes structural damage to the blood-brain barrier, the "firewall" that protects the brain from toxic invasion. Researchers have discovered that obesity in younger middle age may lead to a damaged blood-brain barrier in older age.[3]

In time, this debilitating cycle starts with a high-fat, high-sugar diet. Eventually this kind of diet alters the hippocampus and prefrontal cortex, resulting in degraded memory and an intake-regulation system that's on the blink. In the face of fast-food establishments that provide free refills and giant orders of fries, trouble ensues. The eat-overeat cycle continues with ever-worsening results.

Research indicates that even healthy 19- to 28-year-old men who consumed a diet high in saturated fats had significantly decreased attention spans and slower mental processing speeds for up to five days after consuming fatty foods. And healthy adults (ages 33 to 35) of normal weight performed badly on vocabulary and verbal fluency tests compared to those who ate a diet of whole foods, rich in fruits and vegetables.

And it isn't just adults whose behaviors are affected by their food. Children given foods high in fats and sugars have increased incidence of attention deficit hyperactivity disorder. Most shocking, however, is the actual shrinkage of the left hippocampus, that all-important memory center of the brain, which occurs when the Western diet prevails. No wonder Alzheimer's disease is called "diabetes of the brain."

But not everyone in the world is suffering with Alzheimer's and other dementias. In Africa, India, and South Asia, it barely exists. Japan began seeing an increase in Alzheimer's cases only since 1960, when their diets shifted to include more meat and fewer whole grains. Also, Africans and Asians who immigrate to Western Europe or to North America and adopt a Western diet develop Alzheimer's as frequently as we Westerners do. Obviously, these newcomers have not changed their genetics—just their diet.

The place on earth with the lowest known incidence of Alzheimer's is rural India, where people eat whole grains, very little meat, and plenty of legumes.

As we become more aware that what's on the menu affects what's in our head, I imagine each of us will be willing to make dietary adjustments toward a healthier lifestyle. Sometimes all we need is a few good suggestions to inspire us to eat more healthfully. Stay encouraged and keep reading. There's some great food yet to come!

Eating for Pleasure

If the last chapter was a downer to read, I apologize. Honestly, it wasn't a picnic to write. But isn't it better to have our eyes open to the hazards of poor food choices? We can live knowledgeably when we are aware of the demons in our diets. Conversely, blindly eating ourselves witless is no way to live.

Another way we can't live is "on a diet." I mean a *diet* diet. If a diet involves eating an exorbitant amount of grapefruit or cauliflower or some other fad-of-the-moment food, in no time at all it will lead to an abhorrence of the "wonder food." If suddenly carbs are forbidden and dry chicken breasts are the new it food, in a matter of months most people will reject chicken and rush to a loaf of bread as if it's a long-lost love. If a diet is not comfortably sustainable for years, there's little chance that freshly shed pounds are gone for good. Losing the same 15 or 20 pounds again and again is called yo-yo dieting. When we're told to cut carbs, we quickly peel off some pounds, but this is often due to temporary water loss. This unsustainable restriction usually ends in failure. If this has happened to you, you know what comes next: a gloomy season of self-loathing and shame over being unable to maintain what was unsustainable to begin with.

Deep sigh. It's time to cut out the shame and guilt and be comforted to know there's a more enjoyable path to good nutrition than starvation and cruel withholding of every tasty morsel.[1]

Moderation in all things edible is what works. Tweaking our diets toward more healthful eating has a much higher success rate than going cold turkey on every offending food item. For example, if soft drinks (which are nutritionally empty calories) are the downfall, let's take stock of weekly consumption. How about cutting our soda intake in half for a week? And cut it in half again the following week. Eventually, replace soda pop with sparkling water, and that hankering for a 12-ounce cola (with its 8.5 teaspoons of sugar) will diminish to the point where we can't believe we ever thought it was good. Or if we still adore cola, how about making it a special treat to be enjoyed on Sunday afternoons? Or only at the movies on a Saturday night?

As Mireille Guiliano says in her book *French Women Don't Get Fat,* focusing on pleasure rather than deprivation leads to greater success in keeping weight under control. Variety is also important to avoid the boredom that leads to the return to abysmal food choices. Replacing unhealthful foods (french fries, chips, hot dogs, donuts, store-bought cookies, fast-food burgers…) with nutrient-rich choices (whole-grain muffins, roasted sweet potatoes, grilled portabellas, yogurt, a wide range of fruits and vegetables…) makes a huge difference.

Even choosing a cup of coffee over a calorie-laden mocha latte will save hundreds of empty calories. And when it comes to our much-loved chocolate, let's trade a giant inferior-quality bar for a small portion of high-quality dark chocolate that can be savored and appreciated for its great taste and wholesome nutrients.

Healthful eating promotes strong bodies and sharp minds. And when eating is a non-guilty pleasure, we are more likely to eat what is good for our bodies and our brains.[2] As we gather for meals with others, or even if we are eating alone, let's set the table, light candles, eat slowly, and perhaps enjoy a glass of wine. Naturally, doing this at every meal is not realistic, but when we're able to create a pleasurable dining experience and focus on the flavors and textures, we are less likely to mindlessly inhale junk. And when we can sit down to eat with family and friends, all the better. At those times, I hope we will listen to each other deeply and appreciate the goodness of the table, a goodness that remains with us long after we've pushed in our chairs and washed the dishes.

In addition to enjoying healthful food, let's take a peek at traditional diets and their influence on health. As we look beyond our borders, we see indigenous people groups around the globe eating their uniquely traditional foods. Icelanders enjoy a diet rich in haddock, cod, herring, salmon, lean young lamb, dark rye bread, and their lovely version of yogurt called *skyr*. Their abundance of fresh fish provides plenty of omega-3 fatty acids, which keeps the hearty Icelanders happy through short and sunny summers and interminably long and dark winters.

Even when the shy winter sun shines for only five hours each day, these fish-loving Icelanders rarely suffer with seasonal affective disorder (SAD)—less than half as frequently as others who get oodles of hours under the sun. Their diet works for them. The same goes for the Africans who eat loads of root vegetables and whole grains. Compared to Americans, they have very few cases of dementia, heart disease, dental cavities, and cancer. In rural India, where dementia is practically nonexistent, the normal diet is rich in turmeric, legumes, rice, and meat. Still, it's not easy to duplicate the diet of India, Cameroon, or even Iceland here in the United States. Sad to say, statistics show that as Indians, Africans, Japanese, and even Icelanders adopt the Western diet, they quickly catch up to us in size and incidence of cardiovascular disease, diabetes, and dementia.

Once again, we see that genetics is overshadowed by what we put in our mouths.

Needless to say, Westerners could learn some valuable lessons about traditional diets from places in the world where food is less plentiful but has greater nutritional value. One traditional diet in particular, the Mediterranean diet, known for its salubrious dishes brimming with beautiful flavors, is easily adopted on our shores. There is hope for us after all, in discovering cuisine that promotes lifelong physical and mental health, and this approach is more effective than a low-fat diet. It's a lot more delicious too.

The Beautiful
Mediterranean Diet

The first time I ordered an authentic Greek salad, I was taken aback. Fortunately, the white china plate had sloping edges to contain the sea of olive oil with its islands of tomato chunks, cucumber wheels, feta cheese, olives, and lettuce. Dumbstruck by the volume of oil, I tentatively forked a plump olive, and brought it to my mouth, careful to avoid dripping on my dress. And then I tasted heaven. My naive eyes opened wide in amazement. My first briny taste of Mediterranean cuisine was love at first bite.

Populations that ring the Mediterranean Sea are culinarily blessed. Under plentiful sunshine grow loads of tomatoes, olives, herbs, nuts, citrus fruits, dates, figs, peppers, and other fruits and vegetables. The Mediterranean diet includes plenty of whole grains, seeds, beans, and moderate to small amounts of animal proteins in the form of fish, lamb, poultry, yogurt, and eggs. Add a modest glass of wine, and we have the makings of a healthful and utterly delicious diet.

Besides offering myriad ingredients, Mediterranean cuisine majors in freshness, keeping produce close to its natural form, or in other words, minimally processed (with one exception, which I will explain soon).

The main food source is plants. Food journalist Michael Pollan agrees with this plant-based philosophy. In his book *In Defense of Food*, his ideas on healthful eating boil down to one pithy nugget of truth: "Eat food. Not too much. Mostly plants!"[1] I couldn't agree more, and Mediterranean cooks concur.

It is not completely clear why people who eat Mediterranean style have better cholesterol profiles, lower blood pressure, less inflammation, and increased antioxidant levels—all of which support better brain health. But they do. A recent study in Scotland used an MRI to discover that 401 people in their early seventies who ate Mediterranean style for three years maintained brain volume better than a control group who didn't. Also, those who adhered closest to the Mediterranean diet retained the most brain volume. Amounts of gray matter and thickness of the cerebral cortex were not impacted by the dietary change, but overall brain volume was. This is a significant finding since the aging process causes us to lose brain cells, which in turn decreases the size, or overall volume, of the brain.[2]

So what's in the Mediterranean diet and what isn't? Fiber plays a starring role. In this diet, fiber is provided by brown rice; beans such as cannellini, navy, kidney, and chickpeas; lentils; and barley. Beans are a fantastic source of protein, vitamins, minerals, and antioxidants.[3] Plus, when combined with other whole grains like faro or barley, they add a smooth, luxurious mouth-feel to any dish. Stir a bowl of cooked brown rice together with a can of cannellini beans, some chopped red onion, minced garlic, sun-dried tomatoes, a few favorite herbs, and olive oil. Add some chunked feta cheese and some salt and pepper, and you have a satisfying dish. It works well as an entrée, placed smack-dab in the center of the plate, or on the side next to a hearty protein.

This is classic Mediterranean eating at its best. No refined sugars, no white flour or white rice, no hydrogenated fats, nothing fried. It's just whole, real foods that pack a punch in flavor and nutrition.[4]

Getting back to my first oily Greek salad, I noted its beauty and great taste, but I missed its best feature—the wise marriage of tomatoes and olive oil. Ripe tomatoes are rich in vitamins, fiber, and a red carotene called lycopene. This powerhouse nutrient fights cancers and the free radicals that threaten to harm our bodies' cellular structures. Olive oil is a good fat (yes, we need some fat), and when eaten with tomatoes, it increases the absorption of lycopene. I've been happily drizzling olive oil on tomato slices ever since.

Another fantastic gift of the generous tomato is its ability to stand up to cooking without losing its nutritional value. Lots of other vegetables require gentle cooking, or are better eaten raw, to retain their vitamins and minerals, but not tomatoes. Feel free to simmer a sauce or even use minimally processed tomato paste. Rest assured you're still getting the benefit of tomatoes' rich nutrients.

Another noteworthy, nutrient-dense ingredient in the Mediterranean diet is nuts. Walnuts, for example, will improve your memory, decrease inflammation, and lower both blood pressure and cholesterol.[5] Plus, nuts are high in the healthy omega-3 fatty acids that our bodies need. In the Mediterranean diet, walnuts, almonds, hazelnuts, pecans, pine nuts, pistachios, and macadamia nuts are all favored for their generous levels of protein, good fats, and flavor. A small handful of nuts is a satisfying snack. Just don't go crazy with them if weight is a concern.

All things considered, the Mediterranean diet is better at controlling weight than low-fat diets.[6] Fortunately for those of us who live in North America, we have easy access to the same wonderful ingredients that come from the Mediterranean.

And remember, the *celebration* of flavors (rather than deprivation) encourages healthful eating. No other diet gets so many points for decreasing the risk of cancer, diabetes, and hypertension. This is good news for every part of the body, from the top of our brains to the tips of our toes.

MEDITERRANEAN BARLEY AND ARUGULA SALAD

1 cup hulled barley* soaked overnight in 3 cups water,
    or 1 cup pearled barley
1 cup packed arugula leaves
1 cup red bell pepper, diced
¼ cup sun-dried tomatoes, chopped
1 (15½ oz.) can chickpeas, drained and rinsed
½ red onion, finely chopped
3 T. fresh lemon juice
½ tsp. salt
¼ tsp. crushed red pepper
3 T. extra-virgin olive oil
½ cup chopped walnuts

Rinse the soaked and hulled barley. Place in a saucepan and simmer, with the pan lid slightly askew, in 3 cups of water for 45 minutes, or until toothsome but tender. Drain. Combine barley, arugula, bell pepper, tomatoes, chickpeas, and onion in a large bowl. Place lemon juice and salt in a small mixing bowl. Whisk to dissolve salt. Add crushed red pepper and olive oil, and whisk to combine. Drizzle over barley mixture and toss. Taste and adjust seasonings, if needed. Arrange salad in a serving bowl and top with walnuts.

Serves 6 as a side dish.

This salad is a nice accompaniment to fish or seafood that has been grilled with lemon and herbs.

---

* Hulled barley, (sometimes called unhulled barley) has been minimally processed and is most nutritious. However, it requires an overnight soak. Pearled barley, which has had the germ layer removed, requires just a 40-minute simmer but no soaking. It is just as tasty but not quite as nutrient rich. Still, I use it if I have forgotten to plan ahead.

Welcome, Omega-3s

If the debate about healthy fat versus unhealthy fat has you spinning in a Tilt-A-Whirl of confusion, you are in good company. And just as we need momentary pauses between those neck-straining spins, let's take a deep breath and consider the facts about two noteworthy dietary fats: omega-3 versus omega-6 fatty acids. Both of these are called essential fatty acids because our bodies cannot produce them. We get them from the food we eat.

Our bodies need fat to absorb the fat-soluble vitamins that ensure the health of our skin, hair, and brain—and to protect us from many illnesses. But not all fats are the same. Hydrogenated oils and trans fats, which appear in margarine and most commercially fried foods, should be avoided. They are the "bad fats" that increase the prevalence of cardiovascular disease by clogging arteries. This impairs our blood flow and increases our risk of heart attack and stroke.

Going deeper, we learn that we need two grams of essential omega-6 fatty acids for every gram of omega-3 fatty acids to keep our bodies in balance. Unfortunately, most Americans do not consume enough of the latter. Omega-3 fatty acids appear in two forms, eicosapentaenoic, (EPA) and the most important, docosahexaenoic (DHA). These fatty acids are essential for cell membrane fluidity, which has a huge bearing on brain and cardiovascular health. With adequate levels of omega-3s, circulation is enhanced, inflammation is decreased, and the brain is better protected from memory loss and dementia.[1]

Omega-6s are prevalent in meat and in oils made from corn, sunflower seeds, soy beans, and safflower seeds. These less-than-healthful oils show up in mayonnaise, ranch dressing, and many commercially baked items such as breads and cookies. Omega-3 fats, which are healthful fats, are most readily available in cold-water fish, such as salmon, herring, sardines, anchovies, and lake trout. Fish is called "brain food" because its copious omega-3 fatty acids are essential to support a healthy brain. Omega-3 fats are also found in grass-fed beef, wild game, and eggs from free-range chickens (the ones that run around eating bugs and seeds from the earth). Some milk is also fortified with omega-3–rich fish oil. Plants that provide omega-3s, such as flax seeds, flax seed oil, and walnuts, are good to eat, but they aren't effective sources of omega-3s because our bodies are able to convert only about 8 percent of their linoleic acid to the desirable omega-3 fat.

To sum it up, most of us need to consume more omega-3 fatty acids. Most Americans get less than one-fourth of the recommended amount. It would be great if we each ate two weekly servings of the oily types of fish that are rich in omega-3s. But we don't.

It's important to note here that not all cold-water fish are created equal. Dr. Bruce Bistrian of Harvard Medical School reminds us that wild salmon feed on small fish, upping their omega-3 fat levels. Conversely, farmed salmon eat high-protein food pellets that include plant and animal proteins. Both kinds of salmon contain omega-3s, but the farm-raised variety contains more because it has a higher fat content. But this is not cause for alarm. A farmed salmon fillet still contains only half the fat of an equivalent serving of flank steak.[2]

When I'm at the fish counter in the grocery store, I purchase salmon that looks good, smells fresh, and is affordable. It's usually farmed Atlantic salmon from Norway, but occasionally, it might be wild Alaskan. Thanks to the higher fat content in the farmed fish, it is the most tender and doesn't dry out during cooking. If you splurge on wild, use care to cook it minimally to maintain moisture.

Nutritionists recommend we eat two servings of fish each week. But mercury levels in some fish are worth a word of caution. Pregnant or nursing mothers (and small children) should avoid the following types of fish: marlin, king mackerel, shark, swordfish, orange roughy, tilefish, and ahi tuna. Also, when choosing canned tuna, know that "chunk light" or skipjack is a better choice than solid albacore. In addition to being much lower in mercury, it is moist and requires less mayonnaise if you're using it to make tuna salad.

Another good way to ensure you're getting an adequate supply of omega-3 fatty acids is to add a fish oil supplement to your daily routine. Talk with your physician about an appropriate dose based on your diet and overall health. If you are a herring lover, for example, you probably need a lower dose of this supplement.

When choosing this or any supplement, be a smart shopper. Read the tiny print on the labels. With fish oil, for example, find the total amount of omega-3 fatty acids in *each capsule*. This number will probably be different from the number on the front of the bottle, so read carefully. Also, keep in mind that the most expensive fish oil supplements may not be the best. The little numbers count.[3]

In addition to taking a good fish oil supplement, there's nothing like enjoying a delicious piece of salmon for supper. Especially when a piece of fish shares the plate with a pile of greens and roasted vegetables, it's a scrumptious treat for our taste buds, and it's good for our brains to boot.

FRESH HERB-ROASTED SALMON

2 to 3 T. extra-virgin olive oil
1 small shallot, finely minced
1 tsp. Dijon mustard
2 to 3 anchovies, smashed to a paste
2 T. each: fresh dill, chives, parsley (finely chopped)
Juice and zest of half of a large lemon, or all the juice and zest
    of a small lemon
½ tsp. kosher salt, or to taste (anchovies are very salty)
½ tsp. pepper
6 fillets of fresh salmon (5 oz. each)

Preheat oven to 425°.

Whisk together the ingredients from olive oil to pepper. Taste and adjust seasoning.

Place the salmon, skin side down, on a parchment-lined baking sheet. Pat dry with a paper towel. Spread each piece of fish with herb mixture. Bake to desired doneness—about 7 to 8 minutes, or to an internal temperature of 130° for medium rare.

Serves 6.

Whole Grains

In this era of "good carbs" and "bad carbs," we are reasonably confused about how much bread, if any at all, can stay on our menus. And what about gluten and its effect on the body and the brain? Does gluten make the cut?

In our world of easy-access cyber information, contradictory "facts" abound about various dietary items. Whole grains are no exception. Yet most nutritionists and physicians do manage to agree on one point: The white flour that we Westerners consume by the ton is seriously lacking in nutritional goodness. That's because its goodness is stripped when manufacturers create those fluffy burger buns and ultra-white sandwich breads. Not to mention processed cookies, muffins, cakes, donuts, white-flour tortillas, pancakes, and pie crusts—all tender and as light as air. Many of us grew up on white flour and white rice...and Twinkies.

Don't get me wrong. I adore a delicate, buttery pastry as much as anyone. I would walk miles for a truly perfect almond croissant, and I love teaching people to bake cardamom bread, which is as light and ethereal as bread can be. But these are delicacies to be savored *occasionally*.

Day to day, we would do our bodies a great favor by making friends with heartier grains, such as brown rice, quinoa, millet, oats, whole-wheat berries, wild rice, barley, rye, and buckwheat. (Buckwheat, incidentally, is a fruit seed and not a grain at all.)[1]

So what is the bottom line on wheat? Despite our love for this ubiquitous grain, it surely has fallen from grace as the incidence of celiac disease (an actual gluten allergy) and gluten intolerance has exploded. Let's look more closely at wheat, the main ingredient in most breads. A wheat kernel is like a tiny backpack. The outer fabric of the pack is a granular protein layer called aleurone. The main storage compartment is the endosperm, which is made of carbohydrates and protein, including gluten. Down in the bottom corner of this backpack's main compartment sits the germ. It's like a mighty hard-boiled egg, full of life and the ability to sprout. The pack's zipper pockets, which lie between the outer aleurone layer and the inner endosperm, represent fibrous bran. Whole-wheat flour is made up of all these components, ground together and boasting all the nutrients that each part brings to the table.

But when manufacturers create all-purpose flour, they strip away the backpack's pockets, outer layer, and germ bundle. Only the backpack's main compartment remains. And this compartment is ground into powdery white flour with an extended shelf life. And because all the nutritional goodies are missing, our clever food scientists enrich white flour, replacing what they removed in the first place!

That's why a bag of all-purpose flour claims to be enriched with niacin, thiamin, riboflavin, and sometimes folic acid. These are B vitamins, which are essential to our health. So it is smart to add them back. But this processed flour is less nutritious without the bran and germ, just as our backpack is less useful without all its pockets.

And when we get hungry, we really miss that mighty "boiled egg."[2]

The salutary goodness of whole-wheat flour and brown rice lies primarily in the fiber-rich bran. The two kinds of fiber our bodies crave are *soluble*, which dissolves in water, and *insoluble*, which doesn't. Soluble fiber draws water to itself, slowing digestion a bit and preventing spikes in blood sugar. This helps ward off diabetes. It also helps rid the body of excess fatty acids, which decreases our LDL (or bad cholesterol). Barley, oats, citrus fruits, apples, and strawberries are a few sources of soluble fiber.

Insoluble fiber spurs the digestive tract along and keeps us regular. Whole grains are a key source of this fiber, but all too often, we don't eat enough fiber because it's missing from our processed white flour.

Recently, while tracing my family's Danish roots, I had the joy of working with some incredible bakers on the island of Als in the south of Denmark. These amazing people grow their own wheat, mill their own flour, and bake bread for the community. Upon arriving, my first task was to help shape whole wheat and rye seed buns for the baker's kids' back-to-school night. With wet hands, we scooped risen aromatic dough from big buckets. Its wonderfully heady fragrance filled the air. I breathed in the essence of rye and wheat fields, sunshine and sea. The new technique was a challenge, and I was so off my head with joy, I had to keep reminding myself, *Calm down and learn to handle the dough correctly!*

As we scooped and shaped rolls, I heard how these whole-grain buns first went to the local elementary school. The year prior, the baker (Marie Louise) offered her beautiful rolls for the kindergarteners' snack time. Some parents resisted, saying their little ones didn't eat rolls that were "so much work" to chew. But Marie Louise knew her own children adored these buns, so she said, "Why don't we just give it a try?"

Her rolls were a hit! I believe that those are the luckiest children on the planet. They get to eat delectable whole grain, seed-rich buns that are scrumptious going down and keep the kiddos full until their next meal. With all the bran and germ included the rolls, they are toothsome but moist.

Also, the kids chew the rolls longer, which starts the digestive process earlier—in the mouth. This is what nature intended. Conversely, white buns have no heft. They get wolfed down, skipping the important enzyme process that happens as we chew. Foods made with white flour often give people a bellyache simply because the first step of digestion didn't happen.[3]

Here's a great way to start inviting whole grains into our diets: Start using white whole-wheat flour (which is completely whole wheat, despite its color) as we bake. I add it to scones, pizza crust, muffins, cookies, and tart shells. I start with 25 percent whole-wheat flour and slowly increase to see how the recipe (and my eaters) respond.

We can also up our whole-wheat intake by enjoying brown rice instead of white and whole-wheat pasta instead of the standard stuff.

If you're still not convinced, here's yet another benefit of eating more whole grains: As those Danish kindergarteners discovered, those grains leave us satisfied longer, encouraging us to eat less. In other words, whole grains are better fuel for our bodies and our brains.

One way our family gets whole grains every morning is by scooping out of the big glass jar of granola that sits on our kitchen counter. It pairs beautifully with homemade yogurt and a handful of berries.

SPARRMANS' FAVORITE GRANOLA

¼ cup coconut or canola oil
⅓ cup natural maple syrup
¼ cup honey
6 cups old-fashioned rolled oats
2 cups unsweetened coconut strips
½ cup ground flax seed
3 cups nut combination of your choice: almonds, pecans,
   walnuts, hazelnuts
pinch of salt
1 tsp. vanilla extract

Preheat oven to 300°.

In a small saucepan over low heat, stir together the canola oil, maple syrup, and honey.

In a large bowl, combine the rest of the ingredients. Pour the warm liquids over the oat and nut mixture. Stir until well mixed. Spread granola on three parchment-lined baking sheets. Bake 15 minutes. Rotate pans and bake for 10 more minutes or until granola is evenly browned. When it is completely cool, store in clean glass jar.

Makes 1 gallon.

Yogurt, Baby!

Call me crazy, but when I spend my days away from home, perhaps at the library writing a book, I struggle to detach from my domestic world. I've always loved housekeeping, even when home was just a dorm room with a sewing machine on my desk and baking ingredients tucked into a bin. My heart is especially drawn to the kitchen, where I like to cook from scratch and bake bread, but I also enjoy most housekeeping chores. Even the fresh scent of neatly folded sheets in the linen closet makes my heart sing.

So when I get behind on the home front, I wrestle with feelings of failure. At the moment, our hydrangeas need trimming, a mountain of boots is spilling out of the mudroom, and floors are screaming to be scrubbed. Thinking of these undone tasks makes me crazy.

But one thing that eases my domestic heart is the ability to multitask. Thanks to my friend Paige, a phenomenal chef, making yogurt has become part of my multitasking routine. It all began when Paige came for a visit and brought a wonderful jar of homemade yogurt as a hostess gift. Wow, was it ever exceptional! Now, on two mornings each week, I start a batch of yogurt, which behaves itself beautifully while I'm away at work or running errands. So I am able to accomplish two things at once. And at least one of them is very healthful.

Now, I am not a raving hippie with dreadlocks, but even if I were,

I hope you'd hear me out on the joys of homemade yogurt and why it is incredibly good for us.

To start with, yogurt is alive. It teems with salubrious bacteria. When eaten, it enhances the healthy bacteria and flora in our intestinal tract.[1] Yes, I know this book is about brains, not guts, but the two are more closely linked than we might realize. Ninety-five percent of our serotonin, the all-important neurotransmitter that helps control our mood, regulates our appetite and sleep patterns, and inhibits pain, is manufactured in our gastrointestinal tract.[2] Plus, our digestive tract has a hundred million nerve cells lining its walls. Therefore, what happens in our gut has a direct connection to our brain. People who regularly consume probiotics, which come from fermented foods such as yogurt, sauerkraut, pickles, miso, kombucha, and kimchi, are found to experience less anxiety and a lowered sense of stress. What's more, they have a lower incidence of depression.

In addition to producing serotonin, the good bacteria gained by eating yogurt and other probiotics help protect us from inflammation throughout the body. And, as good bacteria become more plentiful in the gut, toxins are held at bay, making the absorption of good nutrients from our food more efficient.

Plus, yogurt is a great source of calcium and magnesium, both important minerals that strengthen bones and help decrease blood pressure. This, in turn, enhances brain health.

Please believe me when I tell you that making yogurt is simple. I wish I could bring you a jar of homemade yogurt to get you started, as Paige did for me. All you need to do is find a plain yogurt that you like at the grocery store. Read the ingredient list to see what bacterial goodies are included. If you find names such as lactobacillus acidophilus, streptococcus thermophiles, or lactobacillus bulgaricus, you've found your culture. Next, purchase a half-gallon of 2 percent or whole milk. I get organic with omega-3 fatty acids added, to help boost cardiovascular health.

On a morning when you feel especially clever, and even if you must be away all day, this is what you do. Pour all the milk into a pot and warm it on the stove to 190 degrees or until it is steaming, stirring occasionally. Remove the milk from the heat and cool it down to 110 degrees. While your milk is heating and cooling, place 2 clean (and oven-safe) quart jars into a 250-degree oven for 20 minutes. Remove them from the oven and let them cool until they are warm to the touch. Place 2 tablespoons (30 grams) of plain yogurt in a little bowl and add about a half cup of the warm milk. Stir. When the mixture is completely smooth, stir it into the pot of milk, making sure it is evenly distributed. Pour this through a sieve into your sterilized jars and close the lids. Your next goal is to keep the jars slightly warm and cozy all day. I cover my jars with ski caps and tuck them into a little lunch cooler with a cloth bag of rice that I've heated in the microwave. I gently place it on the floor of our closet in front of a heat vent. Use any place in your house that is a little warm. Then forget about the healthy cultures, which will magically turn your milk into the silkiest and most delicious yogurt you have ever tasted, all while you are tending to other business. The process takes about eight hours. The longer your yogurt incubates, the tangier it becomes.[3]

If your day's errands are not going so well and you're tearing out your hair, take a deep breath, and for a moment, remember that you are doing something noble back home. You are making yogurt! Rest assured that by the end of the day, you will have accomplished something worthwhile even if it has nothing to do with your profession or your daily tasks. When you arrive home, pull your yogurt from its cozy place, wipe the condensation from the jar lids, and place your beautiful batch of probiotic-rich yogurt in the refrigerator to chill.

Honestly, since we started eating homemade yogurt, my family isn't satisfied with store-bought anymore. Sometimes we add berries or a little maple syrup once the yogurt is set, but we've found the gentle tanginess of the homemade version to be just right without sweet stuff added.

If you are a multitasker like me, you will enjoy the ease and cost-effectiveness of making superb yogurt. (Or letting the yogurt make itself!) Brain food was never so easy or delicious!

Thank Goodness for Berries

If I had to choose one kind of fruit to eat for the rest of my life, it would certainly be berries. Perhaps it is because they are sweet, but it also goes back to childhood summers picking oodles of blueberries, strawberries, and raspberries in lower Michigan. My grandparents took us from farm to farm to get the best berries. As city kids, we were enthralled with the friendly farmers and all their kittens that wanted to stow away in our car. We picked under the hot sun, scooching along on our buns between rows of strawberries or scratching our legs on raspberry canes. Blueberries were the easiest. The bushes grow tall, so we could stand up under them and grab handfuls at a time. Picking any kind of berry was fine with us because the day always ended with big bowls of vanilla ice cream heaped with juicy berries. Today we are blessed with berries year-round, but there's nothing so beautiful or delicious as a fragrant bowl of fresh-picked summer berries. They are culinary delights that make winter berries pale in comparison—unless of course you live in a warm climate.

Beyond the nostalgia and perfection of summer berries turned into jam, tarts, pancakes, muffins, and pies, we are blessed by the great generosity of berries' nutrients. Think antioxidants! A group of researchers at Tufts University studied the antioxidant content of 60 fruits and vegetables. Their findings put blueberries at the top of the list. This explains why blueberries are thought to protect the brain from oxidative stress and help reduce the effects of age-related conditions, such as dementia. Blueberries are also credited for improving vision.[1]

But blueberries aren't the only berries that are good for us. Strawberries provide large doses of vitamins C and K. Also, their high flavonoid content protects against inflammation, cancer, and heart disease. The flavonoid found in strawberries works similarly to ibuprofen and aspirin in helping to decrease inflammation. On top of that, a study in New Jersey found strawberries to be the number one food to help decrease rates of cancer deaths among 1,271 elderly people. The strawberry eaters were one-third less likely to develop cancer than those who ate very few or no strawberries.[2]

Raspberries, my absolute favorite gem of summer, are a great source of fiber, manganese, vitamin C, flavonoids, and ellagic acid, a potent cancer-fighting antioxidant. Plus, they are full of B vitamins, such as folic acid, B2 (riboflavin), B3 (niacin), and B6 (pyridoxine). And for those of us with a sweet tooth, raspberries are a sweet, nutrient-packed alternative to high-calorie treats that are nutritionally empty. A flavor-packed three-quarter cup serving offers 1.2 grams of protein, 0.7 grams of fat, 11.9 grams of carbohydrates, and 6.5 grams of fiber, with only 4.4 grams of natural sugars (fructose and glucose).[3]

But now for the good news that relates to brain health: Researchers from Harvard used data from the Nurses' Health Study to see what eating strawberries or blueberries did for 16,010 women over a six-year period. The mean age of the women was 74. Because the test group was large, the findings are significant. Women who ate a serving of berries twice a week delayed memory decline by up to two and a half years. Researchers believe the flavonoid called anthocyanidin, which gives berries their deep hue, is responsible. It increases the amount of vitamin C in our cells, it strengthens small blood vessels, and it protects against free radical damage. That's a lot of benefit for something as easy as eating berries a couple of days each week.[4]

If you are fortunate to get your hands on a lot of in-season berries, why not freeze some for year-round enjoyment? Simply rinse the berries and dry them thoroughly on a clean kitchen towel. Spread them on a baking sheet lined with parchment and slide them into the freezer.

When they are frozen, pop them into sealable bags and return them to the freezer. Because you froze them individually, you can take out as many as you need at a time. The following is a classic summer dessert served all over Scandinavia. It works just as well with frozen berries as it does with fresh.

SUMMER BERRY PUDDING (SOMMAR KRÄM)

8 oz. strawberries, fresh or frozen
8 oz. raspberries, fresh or frozen
¼ cup sugar
1 T. cornstarch
6 T. water

Rinse the berries and cut the strawberries into raspberry-sized pieces. Place half of the strawberries in a 2-quart saucepan and mash slightly. Add sugar, cornstarch, and water and stir. Simmer until the pudding thickens. Over low heat, stir in the remaining strawberries and all the raspberries, and cook for 3 more minutes. If the mixture is too thick, add a little more water. Chill.

Makes 4 half-cup servings. It is delicious served with crème fraîche or plain yogurt.

Java—for Goodness' Sake

I suppose all of us at one time or another have been compelled to do something only because we were told it was good for us. It may have been pure drudgery. I remember being forced to eat liver as a child. It made me gag, probably because I refused to swallow it. I used to hold chunks of that gray goo in my cheeks until I could sneak them under the table to our obliging cat. (Thank you, Chessie!)

But once in a while we are delighted to discover that something we love is good for us! Say, red wine, dark chocolate, and (drum roll…) *coffee*!

I could kiss those blessed researchers who vindicated coffee aficionados by proving that coffee is beneficial to our health. We may have roasted and brewed those coffee beans simply for our enjoyment, but what a bonus to learn that drinking coffee enhances our memory capacity. Anyone need to pause for a double espresso? I'll be glad to impart this exciting news while you sip a steaming cup.

Most of us are quite aware that caffeine is good at waking us up and keeping us up. As a central nervous system stimulant, coffee offers a mental boost first thing in the morning or sustains our energy late at night. In this regard, tea, coffee, and other caffeinated beverages can be quite helpful. Of course, they may also wreck a good night of sleep if an after-dinner coffee that you *thought* was decaffeinated gives your brain a 2:00 a.m. shout-out, yelling cruelly, "The server switched the pots, and your cup of java was fully loaded!" One sleepless night drives home the fact that caffeine has powerful influence on our brains.

But aside from the accidental late-night dose, caffeine's influence on the mind and the body is positive. According to a group of researchers at Johns Hopkins University, caffeine enhances memory for up to 24 hours after ingestion. In this study (the first of its kind), participants who did not ordinarily consume caffeine were asked to focus on a series of images. Next, they took either a 200-milligram caffeine tablet or a placebo. Their recall of these images and of similar pictures was measured 1 hour, 3 hours, and 24 hours afterward. Those who received the caffeine scored higher on the memory test, even after 24 hours.

Additionally, the "caffeinated" participants were better able to differentiate between images that differed a bit from the ones they first studied. The hippocampus, the brain's memory center, is where we note minuscule differences in things, including people or even tastes. For example, this morning's cup of coffee had a slightly burned edge when compared to the robust, smooth cup I enjoyed yesterday. Nuances like this are cataloged in the hippocampus. And our hippocampuses perform better on 200 milligrams of caffeine, the equivalent of one strong cup of coffee.

It's worth noting that in this study, caffeine was ingested *after* participants viewed the images. Thus the researchers were able to focus on caffeine's effects on memory, not on the initial viewing and recognition of the images.[1]

In addition to giving our memories a boost, caffeine can help prevent dementia. It also improves heart health and helps ward off diabetes. If all this were not enough, coffee is America's number one source of antioxidants. Coffee's antioxidants help fight free radicals, those nasty little intruders who enter our bodies through environmental toxins and destroy healthy cells.[2]

But we must not get carried away here. A moderate amount of coffee is good for us, but in this case, more is not better. Moderation is the key. Up to 500 milligrams of daily caffeine is generally accepted as a healthy amount. That is equivalent to two and a half cups of strong coffee. After that, most of us tend to get shaky.

As we close this chapter, let's not ignore the social benefits of drinking coffee or tea. Staying connected to others is another vital aspect of keeping our brains in top shape. So if coffee and tea draw people together for conversation and fellowship, that's a good thing. Maybe that's why 80 percent of Americans and 90 percent of the global population take in about 200 milligrams of caffeine every day.[3] From Japan to Scandinavia and from Greece to South America and beyond, people gather over cups of coffee and tea to talk and share life. In countries like Sweden, the coffee break is an accepted part of the workday. It's normal as having lunch or going home when work is over. Coffee, the beverage of conviviality, with its fragrant aroma, promotes conversation and communication. And because of its positive influence on our memory and alertness, perhaps it is the elixir of more *intelligent* conversation.

Healthful Hydration

My wife is part camel!"
This is what my husband says when we're seated at a restaurant and I drain my glass of water almost immediately. It's probably because I forget to drink enough in the afternoon as I work in the kitchen or ride my bike. Especially during exercise, it's easy to forget to drink, and suddenly we're parched. But by the time we feel thirsty, we are already at least somewhat dehydrated. We hear that drinking plenty of water each day is important, but how much do we really need? And *why* is it so important?

First of all, our bodies are 60 percent water, and our brains are 75 percent. Water is essential to life. The all-important electrolytes suspended in our body's fluid—inside, outside, and between our cells—provide an electrical charge that is essential for our bodies to function. Our electrolytes (sodium, potassium, calcium, bicarbonate, magnesium, and hydrogen phosphate) must be in balance so our nerve and muscle cells work properly. This balance is essential for optimal brain function as well! So we must drink plenty of liquids—and replace electrolytes when necessary.[1]

The best way to calculate your daily hydration need is to divide your body weight by two. That number is how many *ounces* you need to stay well hydrated. For example, if you weigh 125 pounds, your body needs 62.5 ounces of water and other liquids each day. That's almost eight daily cups of water and other beverages. But when we are physically active, especially when it's hot outside and we're sweating more, we need more liquid.[2]

Here's an easy way to assess your liquid intake: Note the color of your urine. Has this ever happened to you? You have been working outside on a hot day. Suddenly you realize that you haven't visited the bathroom in quite a while. You finally head inside, and you're alarmed to discover that your urine resembles apple cider. That is a definite sign of dehydration.

Your urine should be very light in color, more like weak lemonade than robust cider. Other symptoms of dehydration are headaches, irritation, muscle cramps, foggy brain, dry mouth, dry eyes, dizziness, an inability to stay warm, muscle fatigue, and decreased blood pressure. Severe dehydration causes confusion because our brains are crying out for fluid.[3]

On the other hand, when we are well hydrated, our brains are cushioned the way they're supposed to be, and our central nervous system can function well as it sends electrical signals along nerve pathways. With plenty of water in our system, our brains can concentrate. We are more alert and cheerful. Our memory is sharper, and we are less likely to experience anxiety and depressive thoughts.[4] With all these positives, why do we let ourselves get thirsty?

Mostly, we simply forget to drink. As we approach early middle age, our brains become less sensitive to thirst signals. This sensitivity continues to wane as the years drift by.[5]

As I have worked with elderly patients (as part of my nursing duties), I've noticed that some of them have an aversion to drinking water. Fortunately, *all* the liquids we drink count toward the goal of consuming at least half our body weight in ounces each day. Milk, yogurt, unsweetened fruit juices, soups, fruits, and vegetables are all good sources of liquid. Even coffee and tea can be counted. The only truly dehydrating liquids are alcoholic beverages. Don't think a beer after cutting the grass is going to replace the moisture lost in sweat. (If you feel that you simply must reward yourself with that beer, chug a big glass of water first.)

Remember that when exercising, it is important replace the water and the electrolytes we lose by sweating. This is easily accomplished by drinking a cup of nonfat chocolate milk, a sports drink, or even a cup of water with a half teaspoon of salt dissolved into it, during and after exercise. (It's also important to hydrate before you run, ride, hike, and so on.)

If you are running a marathon or tackling a similar physical challenge, be sure to get good advice on maintaining hydration. Most side stitches or muscle cramps associated with endurance sports are caused by dehydration.[6]

I hope you are sprinting to the kitchen for a thirst-quenching glass of water! By tuning in to what our bodies are telling us, we can stay healthfully hydrated. If we ignore the subtle hints, our bodies will scream louder with a headache or an irritable spirit. Let's be camels and pay attention to the gentle reminder to drink enough to keep our brains functioning effectively and happily. The rest of our bodies will follow suit.

HINTS FOR HYDRATION

- Remember to begin your day with two glasses of water after you wake up.

- Sometimes we need visual reminders to drink water. Fill a pitcher and set it on the kitchen counter or on your desk. Take gulps at regular intervals throughout the day.

- Purchase a water bottle you like. Fill it to take along on errands, sipping as you go.

- It is better for our fluid intake to be spread out evenly over the whole day rather than chugging a quart right after the morning alarm goes off. Our stomachs have a built-in "empty rate," and that's why we get that bloated feeling when we drink too much at one time.

Chocolate on the Brain

Okay, now for something fun and delicious—chocolate! I don't know about you, but I am definitely motivated by all things tasty. I was born with a sweet tooth, and I haven't outgrown it. But the first 12 years of my life went by with precious little chocolate because our pediatrician convinced my mom that it gave me eczema. I can still see the chocolate Easter bunnies lined up at our house—three brown ones for my siblings and a white one for me. (White chocolate contains just the cocoa fat, not the brown cacao, which was the suspected allergen in my case.)

I thought my white bunny was just as wonderful as my siblings' brown ones. But my sister let me nibble one of her brown bunny's ears, and I realized what I was missing.

By the time I hit middle school, I'd had enough Good & Plenty and other chocolate surrogates. On walks home from school, I ventured secretly into the land of chocolate, hiding all evidence from my parents. I could make a candy bar last for a mile and a quarter, one tiny bit of goodness at a time. These were not fine chocolate bars, mind you. They were basic American run-of-the-mill candy bars that all my peers were enjoying. And even if they made my wrists break out, there was no turning back now.

I began to outgrow my chocolate allergy the following summer, just in time for my grandmother's return from her native Denmark.

She came bearing beautiful bars of dark chocolate, the likes of which I had never known. On first sample, it tasted bitter. I wrinkled my nose and tucked my chocolate away in my dresser. But I kept going back to it, scraping the surface between my front teeth and enjoying its deep, fruity, and almost licorice taste. Before that bar was gone, I'd become a dark-chocolate lover.

Now, many years and many pounds of dark chocolate later, I am delighted to share the good news that chocolate has a lot going for it. It even boosts cognition. Several years ago, a comprehensive study (the Maine-Syracuse Longitudinal Study or MSLS) explored the effects of cardiovascular health on brain function. It considered risk factors such as blood pressure, obesity, smoking, and diabetes.[1]

When this 30-year project began, chocolate was not on anyone's radar. But Professor Georgie Crichton of the Nutritional Physiology Research Centre of South Australia used the MSLS as a springboard to study the effects of chocolate consumption on 968 dementia-free people, ages 23 to 98. As she reviewed the data, Crichton made a surprising discovery. Participants who enjoyed eating chocolate once or twice a week scored significantly higher on specific cognitive tests. They showed greater visual-spatial ability and organization, meaning they could better understand and remember the relationships between objects in a physical space. They also scored higher on scanning and tracking, which is the ability to visually focus on various objects. Their working memory was somewhat improved, as was their verbal memory. This means they had greater ability to process new and existing information, and they remembered words better.

Yet since chocolate's influence on brain health was not the goal of the original study, the food questionnaire did not specify which kind of chocolate the participants ate or exactly how much they ate. Only frequency was noted, but this was enough to convince researchers that a weekly dose of chocolate is good for cognition.[2] Let's consider why this is so.

First, chocolate is rich in antioxidants. Cocoa flavanols positively influence various physiological processes, such as increasing blood flow to the brain. Greater blood perfusion to the brain's hippocampus improves memory and the ability to learn. One Harvard study found that after drinking two cups of hot chocolate, people enjoyed increased blood flow to the brain for two to three hours.[3] A nice cup of hot cocoa, anyone?

Dark chocolate is known to release endorphins, which promote a feeling of well-being. This is why we might crave chocolate in the same way our bodies long for a brisk run after work. It makes us feel good. Also, chocolate contains tryptophan, a precursor to serotonin (the neurotransmitter that floods us with waves of happiness).

Now let's dig deeper into those cocoa flavanols, the primary provider of goodness in chocolate. Flavanols are a type of plant nutrient, also present in red wine, blueberries, apples, pears, cherries, peanuts, and tea. They're good for our bodies because they lower blood pressure, help prevent inflammation, and help neutralize toxins in the brain. This, in turn, helps protect us from heart disease and cancers.[4]

When cocoa pods are harvested, their beans are fermented, dried, roasted, and made into cocoa, which eventually becomes chocolate. The greater the amount of cocoa in chocolate, the darker it is, and the more flavanols it contains.

Milk chocolate packs less cacao than dark chocolate. A standard milk chocolate bar may be only 10 or 11 percent cacao. Compare that to a dark-chocolate bar, which is 72 percent cacao (or higher).

Most research supports the idea that dark chocolate is better for us than milk chocolate. If milk chocolate has been your go-to, you might have to acquire a taste for the darker stuff. Try a 60 percent bar, and once the taste begins to grow on you, bump yourself up to 70 or 72 percent. Part of what makes chocolate appealing is its feel in the mouth, which comes from the cocoa fat content. The higher the cocoa content, the lower the fat. That's why I think a nice balance between chocolate high in flavanols and smoothness is achieved at a cacao percentage of 70 to 80.[5]

Get in the habit of reading chocolate labels. Skip cheap bars that have too much sugar or added hydrogenated fats. And remember that chocolate is a high-calorie and (usually) a high-fat food. It's beneficial to have some high-quality chocolate in our diets, but we shouldn't go crazy.

CHOCOLATE WITH A CONSCIENCE

The chocolate industry is notorious for utilizing child and slave labor. To eat chocolate with a clear conscience, look for chocolate labeled "Direct Trade" or "Bean to Bar." This indicates that farmers who grew the cacao beans are getting a fair price for their product. Most likely, the chocolatier has a relationship with the cacao bean grower and knows they are not subsidizing the price of chocolate by exploiting children or our rain forests. If you can't find Direct Trade chocolate, look for "Fair Trade" label, such as the Green & Black's brand, which can be found in most grocery stores.[6] Fair Trade means that cacao beans are grown sustainably and that the workers involved are treated well and compensated fairly.

Why Dad Should Move to Minnesota

By now I'll assume we agree that good nutrition is vital to keeping our minds sharp. As we stock our pantries and fridges with plenty of whole grains, generous amounts of fruits and vegetables, fish rich in omega-3s, and probiotics like yogurt, we're well on our way to healthful eating. But what gets to our mouths is influenced by more factors than what we tote home in a grocery bag. What about our eating environment? In America today, we eat one-fifth of our meals in the car, and 25 percent of us consume at least one meal a day from a fast-food establishment.[1]

And when we do manage to dine at home, where are we eating? More importantly, with whom?

Family meals, eaten around the table in some semblance of togetherness, have a powerful influence on children's success in school. Kids who eat with their family at least five evenings each week are much less likely to use drugs or alcohol or drop out of school.[2] What happens at the table, around a slow cooker of simple chili, or even over boxes of Chinese takeout, *matters*. It matters relationally, nutritionally, and socially.

What happens, then, to the elderly segment of the population when the children are raised and gone? What happens when one member of a couple passes away? Ninety-eight percent of married retirees say that their mealtimes are enjoyable. But when one of them loses a spouse, that percentage drops with a thud to 26 percent. In fact, half of this group say they eat only to keep from starving.[3] So it's clear that we never outgrow the benefits of dining with people we care about.

Widows and widowers often face the greatest sense of loss and loneliness when they sit down to dine alone. This explains why elderly folks who eat alone consume 2.3 fewer servings of vegetables a day than those who eat with family or friends.

Many lonely elderly people are malnourished.[4] A study that surveyed the eating habits of 2,200 older individuals found that of the 901 who were at risk for malnutrition, 850 dined alone. Additional research has indicated that widows who have eating companions are not as prone to malnutrition as their more solitary companions are. In other words, widowhood doesn't promote malnutrition, but eating solo does.[5]

Whether we are introverts or extroverts, we are wired to enjoy food with others. Food just tastes better when we share it with our fellow diners. This is particularly important for the elderly because of several dietary challenges we face as we age. Our appetites tend to wane because our taste buds aren't what they used to be. Neither is our sense of smell. Also, many elderly folks have missing teeth. Others struggle with dentures that don't do the job as well as the original equipment.

But no matter what, talking and laughing with friends or family makes mealtime more pleasant. Some stimulating conversation or even the quiet companionship of a friend is a better appetizer than shrimp and cocktail sauce. Who wants to roast vegetables or stir risotto for 40 minutes to sit down and eat by themselves? For many older adults who live alone (and this group is quickly growing), supper is often tea and toast, or a toaster waffle and syrup.

After my mom died, leaving my dad alone—a full day's drive away from his daughters—nutrition became his greatest struggle. It's not that Dad can't cook. He is capable. In fact, he has called me for recipes from time to time. He's cooked dinner for friends and baked hundreds of cookies. But I understand how unmotivating it is to buy all the ingredients for a healthful dinner and prepare it for himself. He just doesn't do it. Instead, he eats oatmeal for supper while viewing the evening news. The talking heads take the place of family. He often tells me that food doesn't taste good to him anymore. But if I come to town and fix his favorites (a small fillet, potatoes, squash, and greens), he's suddenly eating like Paul Bunyan. He will inevitably complain, "I ate too much." But he hasn't.

I'm convinced that we are social beings, especially at dinnertime. That's why Dad needs to move to Minnesota, where most of his family lives. It's not that our cuisine beats Chicago's, but he can join us for meals here—and that's much better than facing the dinner table alone. Like Dad, many older people eat better with others than they do alone.

I have this crazy thought that a great way to promote brain health is to provide dining opportunities for those elderly people who are often invisible to those of us who are busy working. If you happen to know an older person (or even a younger one) who eats alone, consider inviting him or her for an occasional casual supper. I can't tell you how happy I am when my dad's neighbors invite him over for a meal. He enjoys it greatly, and he always warmly expresses his thanks. But the gift also extends to me, a middle-aged child who thinks about her widowed dad many miles away.

SIMPLE CHICKEN CHILI

1 onion, chopped
2 cloves garlic, minced
1 jalapeno pepper
1 (4 oz.) can green chilies
2 (28 oz.) cans San Marzano tomatoes
1 tsp. cumin
1 T. chili powder, plus more for chicken
1 tsp. brown sugar
1 (15 oz.) can black beans, rinsed
1 (15 oz.) can red kidney beans, rinsed
1 (15 oz.) can white kidney beans, rinsed
Red chili pepper flakes to taste
Salt and pepper to taste
3 chicken breasts, cut into small strips
Olive oil
8 oz. pepper jack or jack cheese

Cut the chicken into bite-sized strips. Season with the salt, pepper, and chili powder. Brown in a skillet and set aside.

In a heavy Dutch oven, cook the onion and jalapeno in olive oil for 5 minutes. Add garlic and cook for 3 more minutes. Add green chilies, tomatoes, cumin, chili powder, and brown sugar. Simmer 20 minutes. Add chicken and beans and allow to cook another 20 minutes. Season with salt, pepper, and red pepper flakes. Serve with grated pepper jack or jack cheese.

Serves 8 to 10.

WE ARE WHAT WE EAT
(A Poem)

Fill up on the good,
Say no to the bad.
Our gut knows the difference
Between tortured and glad.
Yogurt and walnuts,
Whole grains and beans,
Legumes like lentils,
Plates full of greens.
God in His wisdom
Gave food for our health.
Let the choices we make
Show nutritional stealth.
Pile on the veggies,
Hold back on the meats.
Strawberries and blueberries
Are our new sweets.
We are what we eat,
So let's choose what's best.
Our bodies and brains
Are the place to invest.

Part Three

Intellectual Stimulation

Brain Games

Think back to your childhood. What is the first board game you remember playing? Was it Candy Land, Tickle Bee, or Chutes and Ladders? Games like these are based more on luck than skill, but they still have value. By playing them, we learn to share, take turns, be honest, and accept defeat graciously.

Eventually, we grow into games that develop simple skills, like Operation, Pick-Up Sticks, or Blockhead. These require a steady hand and patience. Next, we discover games that combine chance and strategy—classics like Monopoly and dominoes. My brother and I could play Monopoly for days, hiding $500 bills under the board, each hoping to snag the winning combination of Boardwalk and Park Place.

Ultimately, games of true strategy, such as chess and Scrabble, engage our minds and entertain us the most. To win at these games, we must put on our thinking caps, draw on memory, and pay attention. Of course, if a game is truly a *game*, it must be fun. And isn't it great when fun comes with side benefits, such as sharpening our brains?

With baby boomers' heightened desire to maintain nimble minds, games that require brainpower are hot right now. Every newspaper offers a crossword puzzle and sudoku. And young and old alike enjoy games based on words, colors, numbers, remembering facts, or solving riddles.

To say that daily crossword puzzles will prevent every type of dementia would be irresponsible, but doing crossword puzzles and other brainteasers does challenge the brain with mental gymnastics that encourage strong cognitive function.

This doesn't mean that if you're a whiz at sudoku you will also excel at solving algebraic equations. And people who play lots of Scrabble don't necessarily have better vocabularies than those who don't. But when we tackle mental tasks that use several areas of the brain at once, we encourage neurogenesis, or the growth of brain cells. Games or tasks that involve problem solving cause one part of the brain to communicate with another part.

For example, when I draw a detailed map to guide newcomers to our house for dinner, I am activating my long-term memory, short-term memory, spatial skills, and hand-eye coordination. And drawing a map is a relatively simple task. Higher-level problem solving is even better for our brains.[1]

The games that are most beneficial urge us to think in new ways. When we solve riddles, assemble IKEA furniture, or figure out a brainteaser, we stretch and strengthen our minds, just as we do with our muscles during a workout at the gym.[2]

Brain games abound. Our phones are full of game apps. (If you've perused Apple's App Store or Google Play, you know what I mean.) My husband and I enjoy Words With Friends, which is Scrabble for the smartphone.

I am not sure this game has made us much smarter, but our game skills have improved, and both of our vocabularies have grown.

Games played in person, with friends and family, are even more enriching. I watch a group of women play mahjong at our local community center, and they have a ball! Mahjong, which originated in China, is a tile game similar to rummy. It requires skill, calculation, strategy, and just the right amount of chance to keep these gals laughing. They profit from the rich social interaction as well as the mental calisthenics.[3]

Whatever your game style happens to be, have at it! We learn from games in surprising ways. When I was little, I loved to play Yahtzee with my grandma. It might not seem like a very educational game because each move is based almost entirely on the luck of the dice. But for me, the thrill of Yahtzee was watching in amazement as my grandma added the columns of numbers in her head. Yahtzee was my first foray into mental math. And that time spent with my grandmother was a bit of heaven on earth.

I Want to Live like Harriet

A dear friend of mine, Harriet, is a tremendous gift to humanity because of the way she has chosen to live. Harriet was born in 1917. Her mother died when Harriet was 12, which made life very difficult as she grew up. Despite many hardships, Harriet was a good student. Following high school, she was accepted into the nursing program at Asbury Hospital in Minneapolis. But times were tough, and because she lacked the five-cent fare to ride the streetcar to the hospital, Harriet had to set that dream aside.

Instead she worked as a waitress at a drugstore within walking distance of her home. This job didn't pay very much, but it offered other advantages. Harriet could bring home leftover food to her family. Best of all, the pharmacist's handsome son, Jim, offered to walk her home after work.

Those walks were the highlight of Harriet's day, and their friendship grew into a deeply loving relationship. Within five years, she and Jim were married. Happy years followed, as Jim and Harriet started their family with two healthy babies, a boy and a girl. This was a dream come true for Harriet, and in her midforties, she longed for yet another baby. God knew the desire of her heart and, at 45 (and then again at 47) Harriet returned to the maternity ward. She emerged both times holding pink bundles of joy in her arms. Harriet was delighted with her abundant family of three daughters and a son.

Harriet had plenty to keep her busy, but she decided to take a job with a direct-sales company called Princess House, which features products for the home. The job gave her some social interaction and also provided extra income for her family.

But as Jim approached his fiftieth birthday, he became seriously ill. Doctors told Harriet he would not last more than five years. Though deeply grieved, Harriet did not waste time preparing to be a single mother. She immediately increased her workload with Princess House. She worked incredibly hard, often hosting two buying parties a day. Although her full schedule was taxing, she discovered that she was good at what she did. Jim was worried that this new endeavor would exhaust Harriet, but she cleverly told Jim her job was "fun and games." It was, in fact, exhausting, but she stuck it out, knowing she would soon be the family's sole breadwinner.

As the doctors predicted, Jim soon died, leaving Harriet with a broken heart and a load of responsibility. But she excelled at her job, eventually becoming her company's top salesperson. With her bright personality and can-do attitude, Harriet was a great success. She raised 4 children and worked until she could retire comfortably at the age of 67.

In retirement, Harriet enjoyed travel, an active social life, exercise, her church, and investing in her grandchildren. One day, ten years after retiring, Harriet received a phone call from a new leader at Princess House. This new CEO invited Harriet to return as a consultant and mentor for the sales team. What a brilliant move for the company! Harriet came back to work, and sales soared.

What fun it is now to see Harriet still going strong. At 99 she continues to work, encouraging and instructing young salespeople. She calls sales reps across the country from eight to noon every weekday, beginning in the east and working her way west through the time zones. Next she has a bite of lunch and takes a little nap. Two or three days a week she spends afternoons at the gym, where her trainer leads her exercise routine in the warm pool. Often, Harriet goes out for a bowl of soup and salad before returning home to watch the news, phone her family, and read before bed.

One can't help admiring Harriet for the way she so beautifully embraces life, even when circumstances are hard. She is a wonderful example of what it means to stay vitally connected with others and to be engaged in the world. She is always interested in other people. She doesn't talk about her aches and pains and what doesn't work as well as it used to. She chooses to live for others. In return, she lives very well herself. She is known to say, "How could I be so fortunate? God is *so* good! Lucky, lucky me!"

Some might say Harriet is simply the fortunate recipient of good genes. Strong genes may indeed be on her side, but she also makes wise choices that keep her body and her brain flexible and functioning incredibly well. She chooses to eat healthfully, keep physically active, maintain friendships that focus on others, and pray a lot. Her faith, her commitment to relationships, and her lifestyle promote brain health. Harriet is always willing to learn new things. She is an avid reader, and on those days when her eyes are not up to reading, she likes to listen to books on CD.

Last year, Harriet was the honored keynote speaker at a conference for young sales teams. How inspiring for the audience to sense her vitality, wisdom, warmth, and grace. When Harriet gets up to speak, people 60 years her junior sit up and pay attention to this brilliant woman, who has a strong countenance and sound mind.

No Pain, No Gain

How natural it is for most of us to stick with familiar activities and routines, the things that make us feel most comfortable. As creatures of habit, we tend to pick the same seat at the dinner table, drive the same route home from work, order the same food off a well-known menu, and play the same old games on our phones. We follow our favorite newspaper columnists and bloggers. We read books by familiar authors and walk the dog on that same well-worn path, day after day. We wear our favorite slippers until they are falling apart, and our favorite cozy chair tends to take on our shape, if you know what I mean.

At this point, you might feel yourself mentally defending every comfortable routine, afraid of what I might say next. Have no fear; I, too, favor comfort and familiarity. Like most people, I choose to curl up in the same corner of the couch, to wear my most-loved sweater, and to park myself at my favorite table in our local coffee shop. I have my favorite authors and choose to read and reread a much-loved Psalm that has been a close friend for years. Very rarely do I say, "Out with the old, and in with the new." But I do say, "Let's throw our arms wide open to welcome newness in our lives." And while we're at it, let's invite opportunities that are completely different from anything we have thought about before.

A fascinating study at the University of Texas encourages us to learn new and mentally challenging skills in order to improve memory and stimulate cognition. In this study, 100 adults ages 60 to 90 spent 15 hours a week learning something completely new. Another 100 adults engaged in activities that required thinking—but did not stretch their brains to new levels. Their minds were occupied, but they stuck with less-challenging activities, such as crossword puzzles.

The study revealed that the people who had to think critically in unfamiliar mental territory showed marked improvement in memory, even a year later. (This was not the case with the control group.)

And the more difficult the newly achieved skill, the greater the memory benefit. For example, one test group studied digital photography and Photoshop. Another learned to play the piano. The neuroscientists who led this study firmly believe that new, mind-challenging activities that provide wide social and mental stimulation offer tremendous benefits for our brains.[1]

This evidence reminds me of Ruth, an incredible woman our whole family loves. Although Ruth is 92 years old, she whips out her smartphone to text a grandchild almost as fast as the grandchildren themselves. She uses her phone to keep track of 6 grandkids and 14 great-grandchildren, not to mention many friends. Ruth is not intimidated by Facebook, FaceTime, or text messaging. Just a few years ago, she wisely looked around and realized that the younger members of her family stay in touch via technology, and she wasn't going to be left behind. She bought a computer, a smartphone, and a tablet and learned to use them.

So was Ruth sharp and therefore became proficient at using her tablet and smartphone? Or is Ruth's mind clear as a bell *because* she took the time to acquire new skills? It's impossible to say for sure, but either way, she clearly benefits from her efforts to get cozy with technology.

And what fun her new skills provide! On any given day, she FaceTimes with her granddaughter and great-grandson who live in Paris. She receives real-time prayer requests from grandchildren. She frequently logs on to her church's website to keep up with what's going on, and she is very comfortable communicating by e-mail. All this goodness is possible because Ruth was willing to face a steep learning curve. She admits that she was intimidated when she bought her first computer and smartphone. But she was brave enough to stick with it, and she is wise enough to consult the experts—her grandkids and great-grandkids—when she needs technical support.

Staying connected with her family is a huge blessing for Ruth and for those delightful children who are extremely proud of their tech-savvy grandma. Imagine how wonderfully encouraging it is for Ruth's grandkids and great-grands to receive her texts, reminding them of her love and support. The new technology helps Ruth remember these young ones during finals or any time they need prayer.

Yes, things feel good the way they have always been. But I bet we could all think of something completely new we would like to learn. It could be just the thing to challenge our brains a bit, to sharpen our wits, even if that sharpening involves some hard work. I can still hear a certain swim coach yelling from the side of the pool, "Come on, swimmers! No pain, no gain!" The same is true for building mental stamina.

In Favor of Memorizing

As little children, the first bits of information we're required to memorize are probably our address and telephone number. We need to know these to be safe. They help us find our way home. For many of us, our first address is etched on our brains for life.

Next, we worked to master the alphabet, enabling us to read. Numbers followed as we began to understand the basics of mathematics.

If you are like most students, you probably hated rote memorization, that terribly dry technique used by so many teachers back in the day.

The rote method is popular even today because it is easy to test students on tedious lists of dates and places. History and social studies lessons often neglect to contextualize events in relation to other things happening in the world. Standardized tests drive memorization of facts and dates. We shove isolated nuggets into our short-term memory bank just long enough to regurgitate them on a test. When this happens, critical thinking is absent. (Also absent is any interest in the real people whose colorful and fascinating lives remain obscured behind lists of names, dates, and places.)

This is why rote memorization has been falling from educational favor in recent years. This is understandable, but the pendulum may be swinging back the other direction once again as the value of memorization is being recognized in a new light. After all, if we didn't bother to memorize *some* things, we would miss the building blocks necessary for further learning. How would one master a foreign language without committing new words to memory? And how impractical would it be for an orthopedic surgeon to not know the names of hundreds of bones and muscles in the human body?

We must be able to manipulate ideas and think critically, but repetition and drills have their place.

As teens, we are motivated to memorize the rules of the road so we can be licensed drivers. In all kinds of professions, oodles of facts are committed to memory. Sometimes we *choose* to memorize something. And at other times, thanks to good old repetition, words, ideas, or mission statements become embedded in our long-term memories organically.

For a moment, let's consider what intentional memorization can do for our brains. When researchers in Ireland enrolled a group of healthy adults ages 55 to 70 in an intensive six-week experience of memorization, the subjects enjoyed metabolic alterations in the brain and improved ability to recollect events.

But that improvement in memory did not appear immediately after the six weeks of intense memorization. Only after a six-week rest period did improvement in verbal and episodic memory emerge. At this time, researchers used magnetic resonance spectroscopy (MRS) to look at the left posterior area of the hippocampus, the brain's short-term memory center. What they discovered was amazing. They were able to see chemicals that correlate with increased memory. Every person in the study showed improvement in memory.[1]

Setting science aside, let's think about the practical aspect of committing words or ideas to memory. What does it mean to place words resolutely in our head in such a way that we can pull them out whenever we want?

Consider the long- and short-term parking options at the airport. If you are taking a long trip, you park your car in the long-term lot. This lot is usually farther away from the terminal, meaning a longer walk (or shuttle ride) to catch your flight. On the other hand, if you are taking a quick trip, you might choose short-term parking, which is closer to the gates. Less time and effort are needed to get to your plane.

Compare this scenario to your memory. For example, if you need to remember a person's name only until the end of a one-day event, short-term memory will do. But if your son brings home the gal he intends to marry, some extra work and extra time to place her name in long-term memory seems worthwhile.

Since childhood, I was one of those crazy kids who loved to memorize. Whether it was the capitals of countries or states, stanzas of poems, recipes, scales on the piano, or Bible verses, I found memorizing to be a fun challenge. I especially liked to beat the boys in my second-grade Sunday school class at memorizing the Beatitudes and Psalm 23.

It is much easier to commit words to memory when we are young, but our minds still have great potential for memorization when we are adults. And the side benefits are really worthwhile. If I have trouble falling asleep or need to busy my mind while in the dentist chair, I send my thoughts to a favorite chapter of Scripture that is parked in my long-term memory, and I recite it over and over in my head. As the dentist does his thing, I am digging deep in the cortex of my brain to recall beautiful words that offer comfort and distract my mind. Sometimes it's a few verses from Philippians 4 that keep my head and my spirit in a good place.

> Finally, brothers and sisters, whatever is true, whatever is noble, whatever is right, whatever is pure, whatever is lovely, whatever is admirable—if anything is excellent or praiseworthy—think about such things. Whatever you have learned or received or heard from me, or seen in me— put it into practice. And the God of peace will be with you (verses 8-9).

These words are a gift if you read them only once. But what a lasting gift they are if you choose to commit them to memory! Then they are yours forever.

Music's Mind-Boggling Benefits

I wish you could meet my father-in-law, Paul. If you did, the first things you'd notice are his sparkling blue eyes and wonderful smile. He exudes love and warmth and laughs easily. Although Alzheimer's disease has robbed Paul of many things, he continues to know that God loves him, and he still appreciates his music. Paul is an accomplished musician who learned to play the violin when he was a boy. As a high school and college student, gigs on the violin earned him spending money and tuition payments. His talent also helped him win his wonderful wife. His parents wisely went out a limb to purchase a marvelous violin for their son, even during World War II, when family finances were tight. What an investment they made! Paul's talent and diligence as a musician have brought an abundance of joy to many, including himself.

What amazes us now is the way Paul's cloud of Alzheimer's splits open when good music permeates the fog that shrouds his brain. Music has a miraculous way of drawing Paul back into the rational world. He hears a few notes, which start his foot tapping, and up from his throat come the right notes to perfectly harmonize with a melody. Words to hymns that are deeply imbedded in his mind pour out, giving glimpses of who Paul was and clearly still is.

My husband, Eric, and his dad play their violins together. Eric tunes his dad's violin and gently places it under his chin. Next he hands Paul his bow and positions it on the strings. He picks up his own fiddle, and together they play song after song from memory. Eric plays melody and his dad harmonizes and improvises as he pleases. The first time this happened we were shocked because until his mind went fuzzy, Paul never strayed from the written notes on the page. We watch and listen in amazement as music lifts his brain from the confines of Alzheimer's. He feels released to play more freely than ever before. It is as if Paul emerges from behind bars on an afternoon pass. When this happens, we savor every moment—and the few clear hours that follow each music-making session. Whether Paul sings, plays, or listens to one of his favorite Beethoven symphonies, he is calmer and more like his former, non-anxious self.

Our observations of Paul's interaction with music correlate well with recent research on music's effect on the brain. While it is widely recognized that learning to play a musical instrument as a child leads to better verbal and mathematical performance, it is exciting to discover that music helps maintain better brain elasticity in the adult brain. A natural decrease in perception, memory, cognition, and motor control tends to accompany aging, but studies that compare musicians to non-musically trained adults prove that engaging with music slows brain aging.[1]

Even if adults did not receive music lessons as children, the multisensory challenge of musical training later in life is an excellent way to promote brain elasticity. One study treated adults ages 60 to 85 to intensive piano lessons for six months. These piano students were also required to practice for a minimum of three hours a week. These newly trained piano players outperformed a control group in the areas of memory, motor skills, and the speed with which they could recognize and compare letters, numbers, and pictures of objects.[2]

In addition to these positive results of music making, enjoying music helps relieve stress, decrease anxious feelings, and maintain a healthy blood-pressure level. Music making also promotes good sleep, which improves our mood and general mental alertness.

Even as I write, gentle piano music plays in my earbuds. It calms my heart and creates a peaceful environment in the midst of a bustling coffee shop. Music provides some of the most enjoyable pastimes we have. Possibilities for engagement with music surround us every day. Whether we listen to the radio or sing along with a much-loved CD, play an instrument or sing in the choir, we are doing our brains and our spirits a favor.

As for my dear father-in-law, what a blessing that music remains a great source of comfort for his soul. Melodies and the lyrics to songs of faith nurture his heart and his brain today, just as they have for many, many years.

Journaling Observed

Her name is Adaline, and she is a friend of my parents. When I was in high school, she stood out among the grown-ups I knew because she seemed calmer and more self-assured than the rest. When we first met, she had been recently widowed—for a second time. Such tragedy seemed unthinkable to me. I saw Adaline at church and observed her calm spirit with awe and wonder. *How can she still smile?* I mused.

Then a close friend invited me to spend a week of summer vacation with her family. As luck would have it, they rented a snug summer cottage from Adaline, located next to her big house on Lake Michigan. I was delighted! My friend Linda and I stuffed our duffels with shorts, flip-flops, sunscreen, swimsuits, and a few good books. These were wonderful summer days filled with tandem bike rides, elaborate sand castles, rock painting, playing games, and dancing to *Chicago* tunes on the hi-fi in Adaline's boathouse.

Linda and I loved the mornings. We got up early and raced to the beach to comb the sand for beach glass and fossils. On our way, we tiptoed along a path next to Adaline's house. Inevitably we saw her at her table, deep in thought, pen in hand, head tipped in concentration over a book. The sight of her in peaceful repose caused us to keep quiet out of respect for what seemed like advanced years and perhaps a dreadful season of life.

When out of earshot, however, we yelped and leapt bombastically down a long flight of wooden steps to the beach. Our carefree days were full of erratic bursts of energy and many hearty guffaws, thanks to Linda's incredible sense of humor. But as much as we laughed and the sun shined on us, we mused to one another, "What do you think Adaline is writing? It seems very serious."

Of course, anything less hilarious than *Saturday Night Live* felt rather grave to us. Neither of us knew what Adaline wrote about, but it certainly held her attention. Some days, it kept her off the beach until late afternoon.

Years later, I discovered Adaline was an enthusiastic journal keeper. As a young woman, I attended a conference and found Adaline, of all people, leading a workshop on journaling. I signed up. After all, I had watched her with amazement as she wrote. And what a great workshop it was! Not only did Adaline teach us practical tips on journaling as a tool for navigating life, she also shared her newly published book, which she penned to process her deep grief.[1]

I was spellbound. I was encouraged to move beyond the shame I'd felt over keeping a silly diary. I had feared that book would be my undoing if the key fell into wrong hands, exposing secret crushes and adolescent whims. I learned from Adaline that journal keeping was so much more than "Dear Diary" entries. Adaline was the first person who showed me that writing every day helps organize thoughts to make sense of one's life, especially when life seems incredibly complicated. And that's just the beginning of what journaling can do for our minds and our hearts.

The peacefulness that surrounded Adaline's countenance correlates perfectly with a study on the value of journaling conducted by Matthew Lieberman at UCLA. Lieberman describes how the practice of putting our feelings into words is extremely therapeutic for our brains.[2]

Further research, conducted at the University of Victoria, supports the UCLA findings and adds that regular writing sessions stretch a person's IQ as his or her brain digs for new words in its attempt to capture thoughts clearly and concisely.[3]

Other research shows that journaling is good for our brains because it encourages us to be mindful of the present. As we record thoughts and feelings about what is happening *right now*, we are less likely to ruminate on past troubles or to experience anxious thoughts about the future. As our brains process the present, we lay the groundwork for stronger self-knowledge.[4]

Our minds are often a spaghetti bowl of thoughts, emotions, dreams, fears, disappointments, ambitions, and hopes. Journaling helps us make sense of the mental mess. The process of simply naming a dream or stating a goal makes it real. Written goals are more likely to be achieved. I surprised myself recently by finding an old list of goals that, in an optimistic moment, I'd scribbled around the edge of a paper placemat. One of those goals: Write books. I have now written a few of them. I cannot be sure, but perhaps naming that desire helped the dream come true.

Another valuable aspect of journaling, according to journaling guru Dr. James Pennebaker, is the healing nature of expressive writing.[5] As Adaline discovered, writing through her grief and the many moods it evoked enabled her to face the pain head-on rather than stuffing it away—which could have held her captive to its ferocious darkness. Yes, she waded through deep sadness, but by writing she discovered healing and wholeness, which she passed along to others.

Dr. Pennebaker also claims that as we journal about stressful events, we are better able to come to terms with them. Writing about difficulties lessens their impact on our physical and psychological health. Also, when we write, our analytical left brain is occupied, freeing up the right brain to create, intuit, and feel. Writing clears the clutter in our heads and allows us to better understand ourselves and others.[6]

As I think back to those summer days at "Adaline's beach," the source of her peaceful nature seems less mysterious to me. I understand the value of her daily journal entries. Word by word, the process created healing in her soul. Her book *While It Was Still Dark* is a beautiful compilation of her journal entries, which she began the day her husband died. What a tremendous gift to others in pain, and what an encouragement to keep journaling.

DID YOU KNOW?

- Not all journals and pens are created equal. Find the sizes and styles that work for you. (You are more likely to stick with your journaling if the aesthetics of the practice are pleasing to you.)

- When you journal, don't fret about punctuation or spelling. Journaling is for you, not for an editor. Simply relax and write freely.

- Choose your own topic and begin writing 15 to 20 minutes a day.

- Writing quickly frees the brain from "shoulds." Go with the flow and don't edit yourself.

- Regular journaling promotes better communication skills. A Stanford University study revealed a strong connection between effective writing and clear verbal communication.[7]

- Daily writing strengthens self-discipline, which promotes better discipline in other areas of life.

- Writing in a journal sparks creativity and increases self-confidence.

- The cathartic nature of journaling helps us solve problems and resolve disagreements more easily.

- Journaling our prayers draws us closer to God and helps strengthen our faith.

On Being Bilingual

Mastering new languages isn't everyone's strong suit, and yet just giving it a try has tremendous value for our brains. We probably all know some amazing people who pick up new languages like the rest of us learn the lyrics to a new song. My friend Barbara is from the South Side of Chicago, and she and I share a few dialectical quirks. Our husbands tease us about the way we were taught to pronounce "Parmesan cheese." If you have even a dash of Italian heritage, our pronunciation would hurt your ears.

Today, Barb and I have mended our Chicago-speak, but she has gone way beyond that. She is fluent in six languages.

As a young missionary, Barb learned French, Lingala, and Sango, which she needed to do medical work in Congo and the Central African Republic. When a civil war required her to relocate, the focus of Barb's efforts changed as she began to interact with Fulani people. So she added Fulfulde to her repertoire.

If you're beginning to think Barb is an adventuresome, brave soul, you are correct, but her story does not stop here. The next big change happened for Barb when she fell in love with Steve, a German-speaking American who was on his way to serve a church in northern Belgium. Once again Barb was on the move, planning a wedding and enrolling in Dutch language classes. (Ironically, Belgium is where Barb had first studied French on her way to Africa, years ago.)

A few years ago, I had the amazing pleasure of visiting Barb and seeing her work in Belgium. Wow, was I ever grateful for her language skills, which eased us through the market, train stations, and worship at her church. Her ability to speak Dutch opens doors to friendships and ministry. She befriends many refugees in Belgium who are also learning Dutch. And while the ministry is going strong, it seems that God, in His wisdom, has yet another new place for Barb and Steve and another new language for them to learn.

Soon they will begin work in southern Sweden, where the craziest dialect of the Swedish language is spoken. It is Swedish, but sounds more like Danish. Danish, I am sorry to inform you, is a language spoken from deep in the throat. It sounds like a goat choking on mashed potatoes. (I say this with no rancor, because I am a half Swedish, half Danish-American. When my father began kindergarten as a young immigrant in Chicago, he spoke only Danish.)

Once again, language classes are underway for Barb and Steve. Soon they will settle in the lovely land of ABBA and cardamom rolls. Goat dialect aside, I tease them that they will not only learn Swedish easily, but they will always be sound of mind because of the mental gymnastics required every time they delve into a new culture and its language. As they courageously take on new languages, out of love for God and their desire to serve well, they receive the side benefit of excellent cognitive exercise.

Here are some amazing facts about being bilingual (or even multilingual). The density of gray matter in the brain of bilinguals is greater than that of monolinguals.[1] Our gray matter is where most of our synapses fire, and bilinguals are better at filtering out unnecessary word clutter. As a brain strains to function in two languages, it is constantly exercising. This helps keep it in shape. A TED Ed video notes that being bilingual can help a person stave off dementia and Alzheimer's for up to five years.[2]

Another study at Northwestern University found that bilingual high school students were better at multitasking than their monolingual peers because they are better at selective attention. In other words, they are better able to differentiate specific sounds or words, even amid distractions and mental background noise. Better efficiency at higher-level brain function is an incredible advantage that one can attain by studying another language.[3]

In addition to these benefits, I must point out the sheer joy of immersing oneself in a new language. For Barb, cracking the code of Dutch opened doors of friendships with native Belgians and with Dutch-learning refugees. This is big stuff. For me, learning the language of my ancestors allows me to enjoy reading Swedish cookbooks and talking with my Swedish friends and relatives. It is just plain fun to connect with others in their native tongue.

As I consider the beauty of bilingualism, I think again of my dad, Bendt, and the big chair where he sits in his living room. Mind you, he is 89. One day, a friend of mine stopped by my dad's house and had a good chuckle over his setup in the living room. She was referring to his chair, which is surrounded by papers, books, coffee cups, and a bottle of Windex for his glasses and computer screen. But it was his array of dictionaries that really got her giggling: Spanish, French, Latin, German, Danish, and of course the trusty *Oxford English Dictionary*. All these dictionaries sit within arm's reach. He is not fluent in more than two of these languages, but he knows the importance of being able to understand at least some words and phrases in all of them. I believe that his bilingualism, born of necessity in his early childhood, helps keep his gray matter intact today.

So let us be bold, like Barb and Steve and Bendt. Let's expand our horizons beyond our mother tongue.

TIPS FOR LEARNING A NEW TONGUE

- Duolingo is an excellent phone app for learning a second or third language.

- Google Translate is a user-friendly translation website. You can use it to translate text, speech, and even real-time video.

- Watching TV or movies in another language enhances learning. Use the subtitles.

- Even if we make mistakes, speaking another person's language honors them and helps grow relationships and expand our world view.

Art and Arteries

My family of origin is replete with biology-loving folks who work in medicine and science. Those who hang on my side of the family tree might well discuss the molecular makeup of chocolate or tapeworms at dinner. We think nothing of it, and nothing ruins our appetites. Nevertheless, discussions of surgeries, infections, and the contents of petri dishes are met with groans from my husband and children.

I married a more left-brained, musically talented man, and voilà: We have three children who all graduated college with degrees in art. Okay, one of them mixed in some environmental science, and one works in a form of design that requires a lot of math, but basically their brains lean left.

Yikes! Did we drag our young ones through too many art museums? Did we promote too much creativity and not enough science? Now that each of them is a talented and trained artist, launching careers is trickier than if they had studied one of the hard sciences. But this is where we are—three for three in favor of art.

That's why it gives me great pleasure to report how important visual art is for society and for individuals. None of us would want to live in an artless world. No matter where we turn, we see the handiwork of visual artists. Every building, garden, piece of clothing, chair, teapot, book cover, and shoe has been designed by a creatively gifted person.

Today, from my vantage point in our town's little library, I am delighted by beautiful designs cut into wood on the ceiling, as well as wall murals that celebrate the history of our local lake community. On the floor sits a colorful wooden boat, about five feet long from stem to stern. It beckons children to grab a book and jump aboard; to take a seat, and read. Standing on his hind legs by the door is a giant beaver carved from a tree trunk, welcoming everyone into the land of storybooks. Each piece was made by an artist. Even at the library, our souls are nourished by creative expressions that give meaning and beauty to our surroundings.

When our children were small, our family's favorite Sunday afternoon outing was a visit to an art museum. From the National Portrait Gallery in Washington, DC, to the Nelson-Atkins Museum of Art in Kansas City, to the Art Institute of Chicago, our kids were exposed to a wide variety of visual arts. I never questioned why we did this, but now I realize we were simply seeking peace and calm. My husband is a pastor, and Sunday mornings are intense. After church we find it incredibly relaxing to stroll through galleries of paintings, carvings, murals, textile art, and shiny suits of armor. When the kids were little, their eyes widened with interest, and they produced a stream of questions.

Today, our children lead the way. My husband and I question *them* because they understand art and its history much better than we do.

Years ago, our subconscious quest for tranquility steered us to the art museum. It was an unnamed basic desire to simply exhale and relax. We went for fun. We went to unwind. At that time, we were completely unaware that looking at art actually *does* have a significant calming effect on the human brain. Several studies report decreased stress levels following a visit to an art museum. One such study, conducted at University of Westminster in London, sent workers to visit an art museum over their lunch hour. Their instructions were simple: Look at whatever art you choose. And they were instructed to view art purely for enjoyment, not as critics.

To a person, these workers reported feeling calmer as they exited the museum and returned to work. In addition to self-reporting, the participants provided saliva samples, which allowed the researchers to measure their levels of the hormone cortisol, which spikes when we are under stress. Cortisol levels took a significant drop after the workers had meandered through the museum for a half hour.[1]

Other studies have used MRI to show that when we contemplate art, the areas of our brains that sense pleasure and reward are stimulated. Blood pressure tends to drop. We feel calmer and better equipped to face the world after we have interacted with art.[2]

Whether escorting young children or simply going solo, who couldn't do with a little stress relief in the name of art? Even when we lived in a rather small town, our first baby's first outing happened to be to an itty-bitty art museum. Yes, she slept in her stroller most of the time, but the peaceful environment and lovely paintings did her *mom's* psyche a lot of good. Art is good for everyone, at any age. From our littlest people to our dear older ones who must proceed with care, may we allow art to heal, nourish, and calm our spirits—spirits that are sometimes too stressed for our own good.

Creating Art

In the previous chapter, we explored the benefits of dragging our stress-filled selves into glorious (or even tiny) art museums. We saw how taking in even a half hour of art offerings can help us emerge feeling lighter in spirit and more peaceful.

Now let's consider taking the art experience a step further by creating our own art. Perhaps you don't think of yourself as the artistic sort, but actually all of us have *some* level of imagination lurking inside our souls. We were put together by the Creator, made in His image. Therefore, each of us has at least a few drops of creative juice with which we can stir up original thoughts and artistic expressions.

It's a bit mind-blowing, but evidence indicates that as we use our hands to draw, paint, sculpt, or photograph (as opposed to being spectators only), our brains experience greater neural connectivity. As we create personal expressions of art, our motor and cognitive skills work simultaneously, allowing greater integrative action in the brain. This complex mental functioning is good exercise for our brains and improves our memory.[1]

One study invited a group of recent retirees to join a ten-week art class. Half of the participants discussed art. The other half discussed *and created* art. Brain scans taken before and after the course showed that those who engaged in making art benefitted from the combination of thinking and actually creating. The parts of the brain involved in memory, self-monitoring, and introspection were stimulated. This decreased stress levels and promoted joyful, meaningful experiences. Even the participants who didn't consider themselves to be artistic reaped the benefits of the course.[2]

I'll never forget discovering the paintings of Grandma Moses at a museum in Bennington, Vermont, when I was only ten. Her charmingly simple style and use of bright colors delighted my young sensibilities. And the way she handled perspective (or ignored perspective) caused me to pull out my paints and emulate her style. But what really impressed me about Grandma Moses was the fact that she began her painting career at age 78. Only near the end of her life did she find time to paint.

Her young years were occupied with domestic service for various families. Eventually, Grandma Moses married one of the hired men who worked for her employers, and she and her husband focused on running their own farm and raising a family. Aside from decorating a single fireplace screen, Grandma Moses had no opportunity to paint until she was a much older woman. She was a gifted embroiderer, but when painful arthritis set in, her sister suggested a paintbrush might be less painful. What a great idea!

Grandma Moses went on to produce 1,500 paintings, earning her 2 honorary degrees. One of her paintings was hung in the White House. Grandma Moses lived to be 101, and her artistic development continued well into her nineties. She is a great example of a person who benefited from the physical and mental process of creating art, even during her advanced years.

Another "Grandma Moses" I am grateful to know is Ginny Graham. Since becoming an empty nester, Ginny has honed her skills as an oil painter and watercolorist. She paints wonderful portraits of her grandchildren, beautiful landscapes, and stunning still lifes. Lucky for me, she agreed to give a friend and me art lessons. My friend Sue and I go to Ginny's retirement community and sit at her kitchen table, where she teaches us about watercolor techniques and much more. What a joy to hear her 92-year-old insights on life and to learn from her skills as an accomplished artist.

As Ginny paints, she seems much younger than she really is. She is a beautiful example of how expressing oneself artistically sharpens the mind. To my knowledge, Ginny has never had a brain MRI after we paint, but I am sure those parts of the brain that deal with memory and stress reduction would show the benefits of her time spent mixing colors to produce beautiful works. Plus, the relational value of spending time together—an elderly mother passing on her skill to younger protégés—is a gift to us all.

I can't say enough good things about the value of making art. And when we make art, we can also make friends at the same time.

BEING ART-SMART

- Our skill level in creating an artistic expression does not influence the value of the experience. (So don't worry if your creation doesn't look as good as you would like.)

- It is possible to *learn* to draw. Some people are born being able to draw, but for most of us, it is a learned skill.

- When it comes to making visual art, start small and simple.

- Rubbing elbows with other artists spurs creativity and friendships.

You've Got Mail!

Can you recall the last time you opened your mailbox and found a personal, handwritten letter from a friend? These treasures in the box, a postcard or a note from a loved-one, thrill my heart. When I receive one of these treasures, I smile. I study the envelope, front and back. I appreciate the way it was addressed and, perhaps, the little "P.S." on the back. I anticipate what's inside the envelope. I often resist opening it until I can savor the experience over a cup of coffee.

As old as this tradition is, the whole idea of writing a message on a piece of paper and sending it across town or across the world still seems magical. Yes, I know that modern technology gives us amazing ways to communicate. Just this morning, e-mails zipped back and forth with our daughter on another continent, allowing us to share travel plans in seconds. It's nothing short of miraculous, and incredibly helpful.

But I am still a great fan of the handwritten letter.

Years ago, when I was a young mother with three small children (ages three and under), my husband and I lived just outside of Washington, DC. Our neighborhood park was a godsend. Our house lay about 100 yards from a playground that opened to wooded trails and a creek. Acres of forest gave the kids lovely places to play, and me a place to find peace in my head. One spring day as the kids hung like monkeys from the swing set, they picked up a playmate named Reece. I met his mom, and suddenly I had a new friend. We frequently ran between her house and mine as we shared life with five little kids between us. Through the years, we enjoyed many play dates, cups of coffee, shared holidays, winter walks in the snow, and summer days at the pool. On special occasions, our husbands spelled us for an afternoon of high tea or a stroll through the Smithsonian. Once, on the morning of a great blizzard, Shelley and her husband brought their children to our house as they headed to the hospital to add one more baby to their brood. Every shared experience drew Shelley and me closer.

But around Washington, the wheels of government keep people on the move. Shelley and her family were no exception. When I look back and realize we were neighbors for only three years, I can hardly believe it! But our friendship didn't stop when she moved to Dallas and we moved to Kansas City. Now, after 21 years, we are closer than ever, thanks to the US Postal Service, which we loving call the Pony Express. Shelley and I could insulate our homes with our letters. It may sound ridiculous, but we correspond by snail mail two or three times *a week*. Over 21 years, our conservative estimate sits at 5,200 handwritten letters, into which we have poured our hearts.

Our friendship deepens as we share concerns, hopes, confessions of errors, heartbreak, encouragement, prayers, reasons to cry, and reasons to laugh. Through writing we can listen to each other and, in a unique way, listen to ourselves. Sometimes letters come thick with news. Other times, they are a cry for prayer, more like a journal entry at the end of a very trying day.

As we sobbed our farewell the night Shelley left our neighborhood, we didn't know we'd be able to stay close. But, in the spirit of Jane Austen and her sister, Cassandra, we found paper and pen and a new phase of friendship that is wonderfully fulfilling. We both tend toward creative thinking, and we both enjoy searching for the right words to express ourselves. For us, this works. Sometimes, when we need immediate prayer, we might text, but for the most part it's our handwritten letters that keep us tight.

When our letter writing began years ago, neither of us could have guessed how important and meaningful our correspondence would become. And we certainly didn't know that letter writing could be good for our brains. (You knew I'd get around to that.) Yes, just as journaling helps us process emotions, letter writing allows our brains to make sense of daily challenges.[1]

Unlike typing on a keyboard, when we form letters with a pen, we are using more of our brains in a more coordinated manner. Handwriting involves three mental processes: visualization, motor skills, and cognition.[2] Both the left and right hemispheres of the brain work together when we write. The eye focuses on the tip of the pen, which we move to form letters that make words to communicate thoughts. It is a slower process than typing, but it opens the mind to greater creativity. Simply put, we exercise more of our brains when we handwrite words rather than type them.[3]

And then there is the aesthetic side of writing a letter. Our personality comes through in our written words. I imagine Shelley can guess what kind of a day I'm having by my handwriting. A hastily scrawled and messy note means the postman is rounding the corner and I know I need to sprint to the mailbox soon. A passionate, hard-pressed inky rant means I'm frustrated. Disjointed, flighty sentences mean I'm distracted or upset. Tears on the page go deeper than words ever could.

Sometimes my dear friend might receive a neat, tidy piece of mail that means I took the time to carefully read her last letter and respond thoughtfully. I cherish the days that allow such luxury. This kind of letter writing goes a long way to promote peace and to let my friend know that she is very dear to me.

If letter writing hasn't been your thing, perhaps start by sending a postcard or two. Postcards encourage concise sentences, and this challenges our minds in a good way. Postcards are quick to write, but they convey oodles of love and thoughtfulness. Why not give it a try? When I send a postcard, I think I get more enjoyment than the recipient. But when I receive one, I feel deeply touched that someone thought of me on a trip, or even while sitting at home. A letter or a postcard to or from a friend is a day brightener for sure.

Just beware—you may be starting a habit that will last for many years to come.

Learning for a Lifetime

The commencement ceremony that marked the end of my college years was typical. It was a beautiful spring day. A warm breeze billowed our graduation gowns as we lined up for the procession. Graduates smiled and hugged. Parents beamed in proud relief. Like most of my class, I was 22, and a young 22 at that. As names were called and diplomas received, microbursts of cheers sounded from various corners of the auditorium.

Then one unusual graduate grabbed everyone's attention, eliciting an extended applause from our class. A 60-year-old woman named Betty who had majored in history and German gracefully crossed the stage. She shook hands with the college president, curtsied slightly, and glided back to her seat. At 22, I thought Betty was terribly old for a college student. But this extraordinary woman was a Jewish holocaust survivor. She was born in a corner of Poland that became Lithuania, was incorporated into the Soviet Union, and eventually was invaded by Hitler's army.

Ultimately, Betty and her family escaped to Chicago. She came from a highly educated family, but due to the oppressive situation in her homeland, attending university had been impossible. Finally, at 60, Betty realized her dream of becoming a college graduate. I admired her and applauded with my class. But in my young and foolish head, I wondered what she would do with her newly earned degree.

Little did I know that Betty would live 29 more years and become an articulate spokesperson, enlightening others with her firsthand experiences of World War II. She was living history.

I share this story to point out that learning is a valuable endeavor regardless of our age. Actually, it might be even more important later in life. Yes, studies have found that those who are more highly educated from a young age are better able to keep their cognitive faculties in advanced years. But it has also been discovered that effort to continue learning later in life effectively improves cognitive function, perhaps even more for those who work at jobs that are less mentally challenging.[1] Learning during the senior years strengthens cognition and helps ward off depression.[2] This happens partly because learning with others encourages social connections, and because gaining new knowledge feels rewarding.

Let's consider the various avenues for lifelong learning. Whether we liked school or not when we were young, each of us is drawn to specific areas that pique our curiosity. We may not be experts in a field, but if we are interested, why not explore it further? Let's follow our passion, think about what we've always wanted to learn, and go for it!

We have a family friend who, in his sixties, finally found the time to join an astronomy club that offers lectures and opportunities to look at stars and planets through high-powered telescopes. He loves learning about our solar system. His enthusiasm for this subject is contagious, and he gladly passes on his knowledge whenever he can.

Sometimes I teach baking classes at a local cooking school. One of my regular students is an octogenarian who was so busy working all her life that she missed the chance to delve into what she calls the "luxury of baking." Now she is joyfully making up for lost time.

And wow, is she good! It's a thrill to watch her, hands in the pastry dough, flour up to her elbows, as she forms beautiful tartlets as if she has been doing it her whole life. She is a great encouragement to me, sitting front and center as I teach, and then jumping fully into the participation portion of the class. For her it doesn't matter that she is the age of many grandmas who are already accomplished bakers. She is wise and not too proud to learn something new. It's easy to think that we should know this or that by a certain age. We can fall into negative thinking: *Well, I missed out on that opportunity, and now it's too late.*

But it's never too late to gain knowledge, to read, study, or under-stand something better than we ever have. Sure, we may have physical limitations that prevent some activities, but digging into an area of study and learning new skills is entirely possible. We must not give up easily!

Plus, we must never think we know it all. One of the oldest mem-bers of our church fills her bulletin with sermon notes every Sunday. She is thrilled to discover newness in God's Word. After a Sunday ser-vice, she approached me with a fresh discovery about Psalm 1. She had read this Scripture many times, as had I. Suddenly, three verbs jumped out to her, giving the passage new life.

She asked me, "Did you ever notice how the man in this psalm does not *walk* in the counsel of the wicked, or *stand* in the way of sinners or *sit* in the seat of scoffers, but his delight is in the law of the Lord? You see, we need to be careful what we walk into, where we stop and stand around, and where we choose to plunk ourselves down." I looked at her in wonder. These words were not part of the morning sermon, but as she took notes and listened with an open heart, God spoke to her and expanded her knowledge of His Word.

By the way, this gal is 92. She has studied the Bible her whole life, but she continues to glean new lessons from its pages. She is a lifelong learner of the best kind. She is humble, excited to expand her mind, and willing to engage in meaningful conversation. She is an inspira-tion to stay curious and keep learning.[3]

SOURCES FOR LIFELONG LEARNING

- Continuing education classes at a local community college
- Library lectures and book discussions
- Talks before a symphony performance, at the art museum, or at local hospitals
- Bible studies

What's So Special About Poetry?

Jack, a literary friend who taught junior and senior high school English for 32 years, told me he is not a poet. But I know better. I received a copy of his book *Garden Revisions: Poems for Gardeners True and Honest* as a welcome gift upon moving to Minnesota. It is both delightfully witty and thought provoking, as are the poems that appear on his website. Jack says the language of poetry helps us grasp concepts in a way prose cannot. Over a cup of coffee after church one Sunday, he explained that hymns are poems, and the thoughts they express would not be communicated in the same way if they had been written as prose. I believe Jack is onto something.

Our conversation made me wonder what happens in the various parts of our brains when we write or read poetry. Research at the University of California, led by neuroscientist Dr. Matthew Lieberman, found that writing poetry has a calming and cathartic effect on the brain. Activity in the amygdala of our brains, which is where we register fear and strong emotional responses, calms down when we compose poetry. The brain gets busy in the prefrontal cortex, our command center for executive cognitive function and brain regulation. In other words, writing poetry helps balance and calm our thoughts. This, in turn, decreases stress.[1]

Creating poetry differs from writing prose because prose is usually more descriptive and uses less symbolism. In Dr. Lieberman's experiment, 30 people had functional MRIs of their brains during a writing exercise. It was discovered that the writers, when attempting to process difficult or emotionally charged memories, found greater mental peace when words were abstract or symbolic, as they often are in poetry.

Explicit descriptions written as prose, on the other hand, increased activity in the amygdala, indicating greater anxiety. (The amygdala is sometimes called the fight-or-flight department of the brain.) When participants expressed difficult experiences via explicit prose, it registered in their brains as if they were actually reliving a traumatic situation.[2]

In addition to writing poems, reading poetry stimulates the artistic, right hemisphere of the brain, the same side that allows us to enjoy music. Our minds respond to poetry the same way they might respond to a piano sonata.[3] Our emotions are stirred, as is the part of our brains that senses reward. The emotional response is also neatly tied together with good memories. I imagine we all have a musical recollection that is connected to a certain time and place that stirs our emotions.

The first few bars of Beethoven's Sixth Symphony (the *Pastoral* Symphony), for example, transport me immediately back to Orchestra Hall in Chicago, on a first date with a college sophomore who later became my husband. Listening to that beautiful masterpiece creates vivid images in my head, both of country scenes depicted by the symphony and of memories of a wonderful evening. Music and poetry send shivers down the spine.

Another study comparing the brain's response to reading prose versus poetry was led by Dr. Adam Zeman, a cognitive neurologist at the University of Exeter in the United Kingdom. Dr. Zeman discovered that the "default network" of the brain, which is stimulated when we're at rest, is also activated when we read poetry. This default network is responsible for the kind of peaceful contemplating we do while relaxing in a hammock. We might reflect on the past week's activities, or on what's coming up in the near future. This semidirected mind wandering is less likely to occur when we are reading prose.

Dr. Zeman also found that reading favorite sonnets or poems activates the emotion-processing center of the brain. These findings are exciting to researchers who are connecting the dots between the science of brain function and the way we respond to art.[4]

As we read or write poetry, the Broca region, or language center of the brain, gets busy, but not as much as the emotional or memory region of the brain. Our brain's response to a much-loved poem is similar to the way it senses a favorite piece of music. This is why poetry promotes a calming effect. It also explains why writing song lyrics or a poem is therapeutic for our minds. It doesn't even matter if our poem or song is any good. The value lies in the creative process itself.

So the next time you hear a song with ridiculous lyrics, perhaps you'll have greater patience for the writer, knowing the value was in the act of composing.

Now let's try our hand at writing a very simply structured poem called haiku. It is a Japanese-style poem in the 5-7-5 structure. This means we write three lines, using five syllables in the first one, seven in the second, and five in the third. In Japanese tradition, these three lines describe a moment in nature. Here are a couple of examples.

Beach Walk
Dolphins deep diving
gracefully riding the waves
hiding in the sea

Beach Walk II
God loves sandpipers
silver seagulls, pelicans
playing in the sand.

Now it's *your* turn.

Title:
five syllables:
seven syllables:
five syllables:

Perhaps you would like to try writing a limerick, which is in the "aa-bb-a" form. The syllable count is generally 8-8-5-5-8.

Example:

> There once was a potter named Bjorn
> whose hair was swept up in a horn
> he threw on the wheel
> splashing clay with zeal
> and he looked like a unicorn

Your turn:

> eight syllables:
> eight syllables:
> five syllables:
> five syllables:
> eight syllables:

Laughter: Still the Best Medicine

Some people have a natural gift for humor. I'd like to be one of those folks who can chuckle in the midst of changing a flat tire on a sub-zero night or who find something entertaining about a canceled flight or getting lost in a complicated city. But usually, I am not.

A few years ago, I accompanied my dad while he endured several surgeries and hospitalizations to repair a knee and a fractured hip. After spending a string of uncomfortable overnights on a vinyl couch in his hospital room, I felt especially discouraged. One night in particular, at about midnight, I mentally wandered into that lonely place of self-pity. Since I was only blocks from my childhood home, I thought back to low moments as a teenager and how my hilarious friend, Linda, could always lift me out of a funk and make me laugh. Seriously, she missed her calling as a stand-up comedian.

I reached under my pillow, grabbed my phone, and texted Linda. Sure enough, she snapped back a bon mot so ridiculous (and yet so comforting) that I had to stifle belly laughs in my pillow so I wouldn't wake my dad. It was just what I needed—a good side-splitting laugh! I smiled and fell asleep. My heart was lighter, and my head was in a much better place.

Laughter is a mood elevator, and it helps us learn more easily.[1] I'll never forget one of my most dreaded classes in college: organic chemistry. Chemistry and I were not very compatible. Fortunately, our professor put a humorous spin on every lecture, which eased my pain considerably. He even included a "rabbit problem" on each test. It went something like this:

> Question: Why did the rabbit eat the wedding ring?
> Answer: Because he heard it was 14 carrots.

These silly little jokes were free points on the test, but they also made us laugh. This helped lighten the mood in an intense class that was more likely to cause tears than laughter. Perhaps Dr. Horton knew that chuckling our way through chemistry encouraged better learning. It certainly made the class more entertaining, which was worth a lot.

Research proves that laughter does great things for our brains on the cellular level, things that help us *feel* better. As we giggle over a punch line or guffaw at a comedy, endorphins are released in our central nervous system, sending mind-mellowing dopamine to the brain. This signals pleasure and reward similar to the comfort and joy we feel when sitting down to a sumptuous dinner or enjoying intimacy with our spouse. Endorphins are types of neurotransmitters that are opioid in nature. They actually help inhibit pain receptors.[2]

Moreover, when the brain hears a joke and works to understand the punch line, it is getting a healthy workout. Researchers at University College London's Institute of Neurology discovered that as we experience humor, areas of the brain that are involved with learning and understanding are acutely activated. Laughter also strengthens the immune system as it helps relieve stress in the body and the mind. The level of the stress hormone cortisol drops when we double over in laughter. We are entertained, anxiety is tamed, and even our blood pressure is coaxed to a healthy level.[3]

On another note, have you ever noticed that humor is most poignant during, or just after, extremely stressful circumstances? I am not suggesting insensitivity in a dreadful situation, but I have watched ER doctors, surgeons, and anesthesiologists who handle enormous responsibility every day come up with some of the best gut busters of all. No pun intended. Unfortunately, most of their jokes can't be repeated in polite company.

I'll never forget a comical moment at my grandmother's funeral. We were all extremely sad to lose Grandma Norma, who had a great sense of humor. Her teasing punishment for anyone who did her wrong was the hollow threat of administering chloroform. During the most solemn part of the funeral, my brother, who had just finished his anesthesia residency, leaned over and whispered in my ear, "You know, she left the bottle of chloroform to me!" I squealed right there in church! Next, I passed the word to my sister, who busted up, causing our whole pew to shake.

So thank goodness for the jokesters in our midst who help us laugh! As they relieve stress, they do us and our noggins a lot of good. Unless, of course, an ill-timed joke at the dinner table causes us to laugh spaghetti out of our noses. I don't know why, but my father didn't find this nearly as hysterical as my three siblings and I did when my little brother accomplished this particular feat. We howled like banshees until my mother banished us from the table.

Part Four

Social and Spiritual Stimulation

Any Volunteers?

I had the rug pulled from beneath me when our last child's high school graduation coincided with a long-distance move for my husband's work. We landed in a beautiful place, but for months I was lost in a haze, searching for a new home in a climate that made me shiver. The prayer I repeated many times a day as I searched for a job and a house was, "Lord, we need a home, and please, *please* give me meaningful work that has purpose!"

Admittedly, this was a self-centered prayer, but don't we all long to know that our efforts are worthwhile? For a reason to get out of bed and give of ourselves? It matters. For me, a vocational crisis surfaced because of a move, but this struggle can be more profound when a person retires. For some, the loss of daily work and the social connections that go with it becomes a huge challenge. Suddenly the role that provided a sense of identity evaporates. Isolation and even depression might follow. This is when volunteering can be a saving grace.

Many studies point to volunteering as an effective way for people to infuse their lives with value and purpose. The surprising results of these studies prove that the volunteers themselves are the ones who benefit most, provided they are volunteering for altruistic reasons. At Carnegie Mellon University, a study revealed that those who volunteer a minimum of two hours a week maintain better cognitive skills, enjoy a higher level of cardiovascular health, and live longer than their contemporaries who don't volunteer. Statistics on baby boomers who volunteer show that volunteering promotes better health. Not surprisingly, healthier folks tend to volunteer more. It is a self-perpetuating cycle.[1]

While it can be a great relief to be free of one's day job, isolation and lack of purpose can be problematic. But some amazing people exemplify the goodness of volunteerism. Dorothy is a 90-year-old retired schoolteacher who spent her career teaching in a school for missionary kids in Africa. Today she lives in a retirement community but spends three days a week helping elementary schoolchildren become better readers. Dorothy bubbles with joy as she tells tales of her students. She is a teacher for life. In her case, it's hard to say who gets more reward, the school kids, whose reading skills improve, or Dorothy, who joyfully continues to hone her gift for teaching.

The beauty of volunteering is that whatever our skill set or interests happen to be, we can find places to serve. The plant lovers in our midst can head to the arboretum or public gardens, where volunteers weed, plant, and water. Those with building skills might serve on a mission trip or build houses with Habitat for Humanity. Is the hospital your place? A kind volunteer who welcomes and serves coffee in the surgical waiting room is an important person for those who wait in uncomfortable suspense. Or perhaps you would rather rock babies in the hospital nursery. Human contact is all some babies need to thrive.

As a retired nurse, my mom took calls for a crisis pregnancy center. She offered a listening ear and hope to women in difficult circumstances. Are pets your thing? The Humane Society welcomes volunteers, as do art museums, homeless shelters, hospice centers, food pantries, and libraries. Even theaters train a throng of volunteers to pass out playbills and help people find their seats. And of course, there are many boards and service guilds that wouldn't be able to give so abundantly without the tremendous help of volunteers.

While people of all ages voluntarily give of their time, research proves that the benefits are most pronounced in the elderly population. It was meaningful for me to be a hospital volunteer during high school, but the elderly volunteers with whom we shared an office probably needed the camaraderie more than I did. After all, I came to the hospital after a busy school day with my friends. Still, my experience was priceless. As a 16-year-old, I loved the excitement of the emergency room. I would hold a child's hands while doctors stitched him up. I packed suture trays for the autoclave. But the adult volunteers were truly indispensable. They served wherever the empathy and the wisdom of their years mattered the most.

Not long ago, I went to visit my best friend's dad. Talk about a volunteer! Bill gave hours to the Boy Scouts, Habitat for Humanity, his church, and various other causes. Professionally, he was a civil engineer, specializing in hydroelectric power. Most recently, as we celebrated his wonderful long life, one of his sons spoke of the many dams that Bill designed. From Paraguay to China, to Iceland and Iran, he built dams that made water move to give people power. But one little dam, in the poorest corner of Africa, was Bill's most beloved project. It was the one he designed as a volunteer.

After working his "day job," Bill went home to his basement and poured over plans for the dam until late into the night. This dam was special to him because it gave missionaries in the Congo power to run a hospital and a mission station 24 hours a day. Twice, Bill went to the Congo. On his first visit, he scouted the dam site and took topographical measurements. The second time, he arrived with building plans in hand. He and a Congolese crew worked hard, constructing forms and mixing cement by hand in wheelbarrows. This was not the way Bill's big dams were built, but eventually they harnessed the power they were after. The lights went on in the hospital. What a thrill for Bill! This was his tiniest dam but his most important piece of work, given as a humble volunteer.

Once again, I am amazed by the proven truth in the Bible's words about how we are to treat others. Philippians 2:3-4 says, "Don't be selfish; don't try to impress others. Be humble, thinking of others as better than yourselves. Don't look out only for your own interests, but take an interest in others, too" (NLT). Research indicates that volunteering, when done out of love, richly rewards the giver.[2] We are to serve others who are in need (1 John 3:17-18). Isn't that what volunteering is all about? Giving and receiving seem to be part of God's plan for His people.

From Zippers to Chickadees

Just for a moment, close your eyes and think back to your childhood. Perhaps to 10 or 11 years old. Now try hard to remember something that an older person taught you to do. It might have been a simple little thing, like how to listen for the chickadee's song in the spring, or how to polish your shoes. Or maybe an adult took you aside and invested in you by teaching a lifelong skill, like how to start a fire or how to navigate the night sky by its twinkling constellations. Most of us learned to ride a bike, drive a car, and perhaps even sail because someone helped us acquire these skills.

When I was in seventh grade, a neighbor of ours was a tremendous fashion designer and seamstress. Because she was the mother of my close friend whose house I frequented, she saw me struggling to sew my first dress. My novice efforts must have pained her, because she patiently showed me how to put in a zipper correctly, by hand. I have never sewn a zipper into a garment since without feeling grateful for her careful instruction. She didn't have to teach me, but she did, and I am grateful.

Years later, in my twenties, I fell further in love with textile art and wanted to learn to weave. My husband bought me a beautiful loom with his first ever Christmas bonus, but I needed some instruction. Through a weaving guild, I learned of an accomplished weaver who lived only a few blocks from us in a house packed with beautiful looms.

She had rheumatoid arthritis, and her husband, a doctor, suggested she weave to keep her hands busy to prevent them from falling into disuse. This amazing woman gave me weaving lessons out of the goodness of her heart. Once again, I am filled with gratitude.

Many stories of older people sharing skills with younger ones make me smile. My grandfather had a stream of teenage boys hanging around his ham radio station, soaking up the knowledge he gained in the Coast Guard. He taught them Morse code and how to solder little wires together to build their own radios. While they played electronics, my grandmother and I were upstairs kneading cardamom bread dough in her kitchen. She was a fastidious baking teacher sharing her sound culinary intuition. Pulling out my rolling pin today still brings her valuable lessons to life. Recently my dad invited his young neighbor boy to bake oatmeal cookies with him, and we know plenty of older adults who tutor children in reading at our local school.

So the question is, what skill will you impart to benefit a younger friend? What lesson will you teach? And to whom? Each of us has something to offer, a skill or area of knowledge worth passing on to a younger person that will enrich his or her life, perhaps for decades to come. And similar to the way the grandparent-grandchild relationship is good for the old and the young alike, passing on a skill to a child is good for the teacher and the student. Both lives are enriched by the multigenerational learning relationship. The brains of both are stimulated and encouraged toward relevant sharpness.[1]

Our friend Mary is a consummate pianist. She too suffers with terrible arthritis that twisted her fingers years ago. One doctor told her to stop playing. Thankfully she sought a second opinion and found more encouraging words. Her new physician advised, "Keep playing; don't ever stop!" She continues on through the pain, which is now lessened, and at 88 she continues to teach piano lessons and play for retirement communities and churches, bringing others lots of joy. We admire her commitment to play and her desire to enrich children's lives by her lessons. She is a great example of strength and endurance as she pushes herself and blesses others.

The Bloomberg School of Medicine at Johns Hopkins University calls giving ourselves away by tutoring or mentoring children a win-win situation. Their study showed improved ability to organize and plan daily activities due to cognitive gains for those who participated in a youth mentoring program. These seniors benefited from their efforts, as did the students.[2] Plus, imagine how this helped parents who are occupied with work and many responsibilities. Three generations are blessed, from the seniors themselves to the parents, to the children who are taught.

It is important to believe in what you have to offer. Is there a neighbor kid whose bike needs fixing? How about planting seeds or tilling a garden or planting pots of cherry tomatoes with a youngster? Helping a child to read is a huge gift—one that may change a person's life forever.

Perhaps what you have to offer is really simple, as was the case with my next-door neighbor when I was ten. She invited my sister and me to pour root beer over scoops of vanilla ice cream and called it a "black cow." We were enchanted. When we sat on her steps to enjoy the foamy drink, she taught us about the wide variety of birds that flew in and out from the woods to her feeder, and she helped us learn the song of the chickadee. Such a simple gift to us. But years later, I am delighted to remember a kind woman who took the time to invest in a couple of girls who had just moved a thousand miles away from our grandparents. Her gift to us may seem insignificant, but it was valuable indeed.

It's the gift of a caring relationship, and it's the gift of learning a life-enriching skill. May we all be open to giving and teaching, enlarging the circle of caring adults in the lives of children. Like many examples of receiving through giving, the dynamic legacy of engaging in a child's life is full of positive possibilities.

Choral Singing for the Health of It

For better or for worse, I slid into college on the coattails of my perfect older siblings. It wasn't exactly easy to take biology with my brother as the teaching assistant. I'll never forget when he watched me mistake the gender of a dead cat on a lab practical. I was shamefaced for a week, hoping he wouldn't tell his cool premed buddies.

Then there was my lovely soprano sister, who sang in the most elite choral group on campus. She was very kind to coach me in singing. She even accompanied me in a vocal audition. But her playing was far superior to my singing, and I didn't make the cut.

As the year progressed, I busied myself with other activities. I studied and baked lots of cookies. But I couldn't help noticing what a great time my friends had in choir. They came directly from rehearsals to dinner, happily singing and laughing together. I loved to attend their musical performances, but deep in my heart, I knew I was missing a wonderful part of college life.

At last, in my final year of school (seven years and another degree later), I realized it was my last chance to sing in a college choir. For some reason, numbers must have been down, because the choral director, to my great amazement, welcomed me in!

Have you ever yearned a long time for something, but when it finally came true, it didn't live up to your expectations? Well, that was *not* the case with my college choir. It was a delightful experience that I will never forget! That year, as a senior nursing student, I had a heavy academic load, and my schedule was tight. But spending three afternoons a week surrounded by beautiful melodies and an entirely new group of friends opened my mind and heart in a way that made the investment of time worthwhile. I left the music hall feeling light-hearted and refreshed even though I had a lot of studying to accomplish before bedtime.

During those years, I had no idea that singing in a choir is known the world over as a spirit-lifting activity that makes people feel happy. And it does more than that. Scientists have found that choral singing treats us to even more benefits than I observed among my college pals. A cross-national study, initiated by the Canterbury Christ Church University in England, found that more than 90 percent of 1,000 choir members in Australia, Germany, and the UK say that group singing increases their quality of life and improves their mood. About 85 percent say it is relaxing and helps decrease their stress levels.[1]

Another study examined the mechanics of singing and notes and pointed out that as we sing, we engage in controlled synchronized deep-breathing, which is good for us individually and collectively. As we know, sustained inhaling and exhaling is an effective stress reliever that helps reduce anxiety as well. But when we sing with others, a bonding takes place. During group singing, our brains are treated to a comforting dose of endorphins that cheer our hearts. Singing works like a tranquilizer that sooths nerves and lifts our spirits. It's not uncommon to walk into a choir rehearsal weighed down by worry, but, after an hour of making music with fellow choristers, to emerge feeling lighthearted and full of goodwill. Oxford University researchers believe that singing in a choir draws people together and builds a sense of community.[2]

Obviously these psychological benefits of singing serve the brain well. But the rest of the body profits from choral singing too. Our choir director never mentioned this, but our immune system is strengthened when we sing with others. Who knew? Researchers took saliva samples from choir members on their way into choir rehearsal and again on their way out. They discovered that immunoglobulin-A levels increased as they sang for an hour. That means that these choir members received a boost in their ability to fight infection.[3]

I can't remember whether I had fewer colds that year in college choir, but I can certainly attest to finding a whole lot of joy, a new sense of community, and a healthy way to deal with stress. Also, luckily for me, studies show that you don't need to be a great singer to realize all these benefits.

So we don't need to limit our singing to the shower or around the house. That doesn't give our minds the same benefit as group singing does.[4] But considering the strong bonds that form between those who sing together, it's not surprising that music is often the glue that lends cohesiveness to religious gatherings and worship. I couldn't help reflecting on this truth as I sang in our church choir this morning, grateful for the joy that singing affords and grateful for my fellow singers, who buoy my spirits every time we raise our voices in song.

Friends of All Ages

As a college student, I had the joy of working part time at a beautiful Swedish import store in Chicago. In a sense, it wouldn't have mattered what kind of shop it was, because the owners, Ingrid and Gösta, were the ones who made things joyful. They were big-hearted, likable, and sometimes irascible. They were a living comedy routine of a couple. I loved working for them. A day never went by without a good laugh, strong coffee served in *real* cups, and the opportunity to sharpen my skills in "Swinglish." Swinglish was Ingrid and Gösta's unique blend of English and Swedish. Words from both languages popped up in nearly every sentence. I tried to limit my "Swinglish" to days at the shop, but sometimes it would sneak out in other places, eliciting giggles from my college friends.

As I worked at Sweden Shop, which really wasn't *work* at all, Ingrid and Gösta Bergstrom taught me a lot about life, honesty, loyalty, industry, and the value of abiding friendship, regardless of a person's age. They certainly had a knack for business, but above all they were *people* people.

Ingrid and Gösta's friends could be 20 years old, 70, or any age in between. The store was on the edge of our college campus, so many coeds came in to browse or purchase a gift or a card. On sale days, they came for free coffee and princess torte, a splendid marzipan cake. Ingrid and Gösta knew the names of hundreds of students, professors, and neighborhood folks. Some students came ostensibly to shop, but they really wanted romantic advice. Both shop owners were generous is that department, as they followed the relational twists and turns of many a couple with genuine interest and care.

When it was finally time for the couple to sell the store and retire, they stayed tight with the abundant flock of friends who had grown with the business. Long after shop days, it was fun to visit Ingrid and Gösta at their home.

On family trips to Chicago, we visited their home for coffee, to talk, and to do what we had always done: laugh and encourage each other as good friends do. Age never matters when friendship is genuine, and our children added another generation to the Bergstroms' circle of friends. Each generation was fascinated with the others. Conversations were lively, covering art, business, politics, books, and what the kids wanted to be when they grew up. Eighty-year-olds shared their perspective on the world, but they wanted to know what the kids thought too. What a gift to build memories with dear people whose friendship was ageless.

Even after Gösta passed away, our visits with Ingrid remained lively. Her frank words about missing the love of her life seemed to lay her pain out in the light, where it was open to healing. She didn't assume we couldn't understand because we were younger. She honored us with her true heart, giving us courage to feel pain and find wholeness in it.

One evening while having coffee around Ingrid's gorgeous modern-glass dining table, Ingrid asked our high school boys, *"So, vot is dis Facebook anyvay?"* Bjorn and Karl-Jon explained that it's a tool to stay in touch with friends no matter where they live. Oh, wow—that struck the right chord with Ingrid.

Within minutes she was seated in front of her computer, flanked by two high school friends who couldn't wait to help set up her Facebook page. They took her picture and uploaded it. Basic information was entered, and her account went live. The boys gave a quick lesson in friending, posting, and messaging. Within 15 minutes, a friend 30 years Ingrid's junior posted a message on her wall. Ingrid, shrieking with delight, said, "Boys, oh my goodness, we must answer quickly so Judy knows I still want to be her friend!"

Bjorn and Karl-Jon laughed and explained that Facebook isn't like answering the phone. You can take your time answering. But Ingrid was in a hurry (typical!) to communicate her friendship with this younger friend.

So there it is—the beauty of relationships that blur the silly lines that divide generations.

On my fiftieth birthday, I was truly bummed. That day, my husband and I, like frozen statues, watched movers stuff all our belongings into a storage unit because we had recently moved and had yet to find a house. I stood by with a heavy heart and freezing feet, trying to adjust to Minnesota temperatures in December. Finally, in a state of self-pity and despair, I called Ingrid to share my misery. I told her it was my "dreaded fiftieth," thinking, *Oh, dear Ingrid, you always come through. Give me a shoulder to cry on like you did when I was in college.*

Instead she burst out laughing, "What? Fifty?! You're such a *baby!*" I was the next one laughing! Of course, to an 88-year-old, I was barely grown up. What joy she gave me with her perspective of years. I was just a bit over halfway to her age, and she let me know it in Swinglish, spoken kindly with a heavy accent.

As I held the phone and thanked Ingrid for loving me, I attempted to wiggle warmth back into my toes, just as she had wrapped warmth around my aching heart. I also vowed right then and there to keep relationships alive with friends of all ages.

Book Group: More Than a Good Read

I t all started with a dinner party at the home of a colleague. To help you picture this meal, you must know that our host was the executive chef at the culinary school where most of us worked. Needless to say, our meal was extraordinary. Conversation was lively, jumping from the glory days of a restaurant to where two of the others had cooked, to books, to dogs and cats, to recent finds at the farmers' market, to the condition of our gardens. At some point over dessert, eight or ten of us lingered over coffee and began talking about a book. No one was in a hurry to leave.

Molly, the mother of a two-year-old, was hungry for more brain stimulation than she got reading and rereading children's literature. I don't remember exactly how the idea to form a reading group came up, but sometime before the candles burned down, five women decided to meet once a month to discuss a book. We agreed that whoever hosted that month would choose the book and cook the meal. I really liked these people, but I felt trepidation about joining. I felt quite sure I was in over my head in both the literary and culinary departments. But I felt strangely excited too.

"I'm game," I said.

I'm forever grateful to have set fear aside, because this book group has changed my life. At the outset, I didn't know how valuable it is to stretch beyond the books I naturally choose. I needed a swift kick out of my comfort zone and into this group of thinkers. Although each one of us has a love relationship with food, we are all over the map in other respects. Collectively we are artistic, mathematical, analytical, married, single, mothers, childless, dog lovers, and dog-allergic. We are introverts and extroverts. We have varying spiritual backgrounds, and I dare say we vote differently. Naturally we don't all thrill to the same books, but we all agree that everything is better with butter, and we never say no to Nancy's espresso or Paige's peach raspberry galette, even if it is late at night.

I realize that not all book groups work out as swimmingly as ours. In fact, one of our members expressed initial reservations because her previous book group fizzled into an ash heap of gossip. We decided ours would be different. With great respect for each other, and with our best intentions to read what is chosen each month, we gather, discuss, and eat very well.

Since we all adore cooking, our meals frequently reflect the theme of a book: Mexican chili verde and creamy flan when we read *The Tortilla Curtain*, borscht for a Russian author, and a Provençal meal in honor of Julia Child's *My Life in France*. It doesn't matter which cuisine shapes each month's menu; each meal is a gift to our taste buds, while the book discussions nourish our minds.

I imagine we have all heard the sage advice that it's best to join a book club with people one doesn't know, or who at least aren't friends. Strangers can be as blunt as the butt end of a gun, and no relationship is ruined in the process. I get that. Or, like our group, you may begin with a handful of acquaintances and over time grow to be the best of friends. If I were dying, I would refuse to leave this world without one more heart-to-heart with each member of my book group. They have become the dearest of friends—over books, over meals, over years of listening to one another, over journeying together. We don't have to agree on every point. In fact, it's better that we don't. Instead we offer each other insights from varying perspectives. Iron sharpens iron.

And while we have a blast together, our reading pushes us to use our noggins for critical thinking. Each month we are forced to engage our brains in the language and setting of a new book. We constantly meet new characters and wrestle with subjects that might have been completely foreign to us. We read widely and discuss deeply. We catch up with each other's lives and enjoy a glass of wine. Social interaction like this increases our serotonin levels, encouraging the good feelings that come with camaraderie.[1] This helps stimulate neural connections that promote better cognitive function. What I thought would just keep me reading has given me brilliant friends whose lives have enriched mine beyond my wildest imagination.

If you have not read with others, why not give it a whirl? If you absolutely hate your book group, simply bow out. But chances are that your horizons will broaden along with your vocabulary and your understanding of ideologies and the people who hold them.[2] Be prepared to get to know the members of your book group, but also, be prepared to gain a deeper understanding of yourself. Self-knowledge may cause us to squirm, but it's how we grow.

This kind of growth is less likely to happen when reading alone. And if dinner matters to you, as it does to me, read with those who love to cook or at least appreciate good food. Sometimes the book of the month turns out to be a zero, but our time at the table never disappoints. It always keeps us coming back for more.

One Thing at a Time

I'm embarrassed to say that at times I've badgered my husband, Eric, for choosing to avoid double- and triple-tasking, as I often do. Many of my jobs have depended on my ability to juggle a half-dozen goals at a time while under pressure. As a nurse, it was nearly impossible for me to care for eight patients at a time without multitasking. The same is true when I have to prepare and serve a dinner for 100 guests or more.

And that's nothing compared to the demands of emergency room physicians or air traffic controllers. In our tech-driven world, who *doesn't* have multiple windows open on their computer? I often think I am being inefficient if I am not cleaning a bathroom or weeding my garden during a phone conversation. So I've chided Eric for considering a phone call reason to sit on the couch and put his feet up. But now I humbly give up my pseudo-hyper-efficiency and agree that he is right and I am wrong. (This time.)

For all our efforts at super-productivity, plenty of studies resoundingly agree that multitasking does not equal multi-*accomplishing*. While it seems as if doing several tasks at a time will save time, the opposite may be true. The way the brain is designed, the posterior lateral prefrontal cortex (pLPFC) takes over when a lot of stimuli hit the brain at once. It's like the triage nurse at the hospital emergency department. He or she must decide which incoming patient has the most critical need and gets to be seen first. The pLPFC lines up the stimuli and deals with them one at a time. Or if the brain is bombarded by too many needs at once, the pLPFC handles the first two while the rest will likely be forgotten.[1] Let's be thankful that our hospitals don't work this way, but our brains do. So we will benefit by treating them accordingly. Because of our amazing technology, we push the mental envelope. We ask our minds to do more than they are built to handle. And for all technology's benefits, we allow it to complicate life for our brains. Cognitive scientist Clifford Nass of Stanford University reports that the top 25 percent of Stanford students have at least 4 windows open on their computers almost all the time. But rather than resulting in greater creativity and productivity, he sees stunted emotional intelligence and a diminished ability to use working memory, which is needed to creatively solve problems.

Nass believes the more we multitask, the less we can concentrate and learn. And we are less likely to be nice to people. Moreover, high-level multitaskers are more likely to make mistakes because they miss important pieces of information as they go about their work.[2]

So what is a fair workload for the human mind? We are not questioning a person's intelligence here. (Though attempts to multitask lowers a person's intelligence quotient by 15 points.)[3] Rather, the key question is, what does it look like for us to use our brains most effectively? Most research says that we can do two or even three things at a time, *if* only one of them requires concentration. For example, most of us can simultaneously walk, talk to a friend, and eat an ice cream cone. We could probably even add pushing a baby in a stroller.

But if, during the walk, we receive a phone call that requires mental concentration, that friend had better take over and start pushing the stroller. When it's in critical-thinking mode, the human brain focuses on one thing at a time. We can add one or two things to the mix, but only if they are "autopilot" tasks. (For example, most people can problem solve and chew gum with some mood music in the background.) Beyond that, however, the margin of error rises quickly. That's why using technology (such as texting) while driving causes 25 percent of our traffic accidents.[4] This is a rather new problem in our society, but its consequences are sobering.

So when did all this crazy-making begin? The word "multitask" was coined by IBM in 1965 in a description of a computer that could run several programs concurrently.[5] Multitasking is all in a day's work for a computer, but it doesn't work as well for us humans. When we give our full attention to a project, we are at our best creatively. We make fewer errors. Or we miss fewer of the errors we are trying to find. (Think of a proofreader working on a book or a software engineer trying to find bugs in a computer program.)

Think about a time when you felt incredibly stressed. Got one? Were you feeling pressured to do more than your brain could handle? For me that moment happened after a stressful day at work. I felt as if I'd solved 300 problems while trying to be pleasant to clients. But internally I was worried sick about my dad, who was in the hospital. As I began my commute home, the doctor called me, and I answered. While I listened intently, I turned right on red where it was not allowed and earned my first moving violation. My brain was fried, and I got what I deserved—immediate punishment. But pushing our brains by constantly multitasking also carries longer-term ramifications.[6]

Researchers note that when mental demand continually exceeds ability, stress results. It's good to have *some* stress to encourage optimum performance. But chronic stress due to multitasking overdoses our brains on the stress hormone cortisol. This overdose can lead to chronic anxiety and even depression.[7] Also, those who are habitual multitaskers (and it *is* habit-forming) lose much of their ability to filter out irrelevant information. This is particularly problematic for students who flip between work and social media, jumping to validate every ping and tweet. This FOMO (fear of missing out) is a unique kind of anxiety that we work hard to prevent by bowing to the constant barrage of tech messages. Yes, missing a text could mean we are momentarily out of the loop. But staying in the know about *everything* on social media comes at a high cost.

What should we do? How about slowing down, setting priorities, and giving our minds the chance to concentrate on one thing at a time? We'll probably discover we are more accurate, creative, and efficient than when we succumbed to multitasking.[8]

YOUR PERSONAL MULTITASKING INVENTORY

- How frequently do I talk on the phone or text while I am driving?

- Which tasks are so natural for me that I can comfortably accomplish two or more of them at one time?

- When have I felt so bombarded by what was happening around me that I couldn't function? How did I resolve this problem?

- How frequently do I flip between my work and social media, such as Instagram or Facebook?

- Scientists believe that we are more effective and efficient when we do one thing at a time. What specific steps can I take to limit my multitasking?

Pets—Best Friends
with Benefits

When was the last time you stared up at the clear night sky and felt amazed by the shimmer of the Milky Way so far away? It makes one feel small to stand under such vastness, especially when we ponder light-years and galaxies beyond our view. It's with similar heartfelt wonder, the kind that takes our breath away, that we consider the human brain, with its tremendous complexity.

The intricate physical structure of our brains is amazing. And what happens at a deeper, chemical level is even more incredible. Our brains' billions of neurotransmitters, sending and receiving messages every second, make us who we are. Our brains guide us through every step of life. Each personality, cognitive makeup, creativity, and way of interacting with others is entirely unique.

The deepest chemical realm of the brain is where we experience emotions. And there is nothing like the comforting and calming joy that we experience with animals, namely our pets.

Whether you are a dog person or you have a soft spot for cats, you know what I'm talking about. Even watching tropical fish swim back and forth lowers blood pressure.[1] But of course you can't snuggle with a fish.

Stroking a dog or a cat, however, provides many benefits for us. Our pets have entirely unbiased, unconditional love for us. That's one reason cuddling a favorite pet does wonderful things for our psyches and our emotions. Research shows that petting a dog for 5 to 24 minutes lowers blood pressure, slows one's heart rate, and regulates breathing. It also relaxes muscle tension and puts us in a better mood.[2] Even if we could invent a medicine to duplicate these benefits, it wouldn't work as quickly, and it wouldn't be nearly as fulfilling and enjoyable.

These outward responses are results of a microscopic party in our brain. As we caress the dog, the oxytocin in our blood doubles. What's more, dopamine and endorphins join the fun, promoting feelings like a runner's high.

Our cortisol levels plummet, and we're treated to a mind-calming dose of serotonin, the neurotransmitter that antidepressants attempt to imitate.[3] This explains why when we return home from a stressful day or a frenzied commute, our stress levels drop as we're greeted by a loving dog who wags her tail in welcome and looks at us with adoring eyes. Collapsing on the couch to snuggle a kitty or pup makes everything better. Research shows that our psyches are most comforted by our own pets, but interacting with someone else's dog or cat also promotes feelings of goodwill.

This is why some dogs are welcome visitors in hospitals, nursing homes, and counseling sessions. They make people feel safe. Sparkles, a dog who visits my father-in-law's memory-care unit, is everybody's favorite. This sweet schnauzer cheers people who sometimes don't respond well to human attention. They reach out to touch Sparkles's fur. If she puts her head on a resident's lap, she has made someone's day. She is perceptive and tolerant, a joyful presence who brings smiles to many old faces as she makes her rounds.

I wish every elderly person who lives all alone could have a pet. They wouldn't feel so lonely. As my son recently explained, walking a dog is the best way to meet people. Strolling with a dog on a leash takes the strangeness out of chatting with strangers. There's nothing awkward about striking up a conversation with someone when pups are along. Walking a dog gives us a reason to be outdoors, which boosts our mood and mental health. Dogs keep us moving, whether it's to throw a Frisbee, take a trip to the dog park, or just go for a walk. They encourage exercise and contact with others. Plus, they make us laugh—another way to encourage emotional health.

And don't we all need a good listener who doesn't judge? That's what I appreciated most about my loving Chessie cat. He was born in our living room when I was 11. He delighted us with his affectionate purring and hilarious tricks. He was my "steady"—my best listener, the sponge who soaked up my tears of adolescence and young adulthood. He helped me study and kept my feet warm at night. And he always met each member of our family at the door when we came home.

He purred his way into each of our hearts, calming and comforting us with his understanding eyes. He was a stress reducer with his thick coat, which needed frequent brushing, especially in the springtime. I know that there are a lot of dog lovers out there, but for a girl who is allergic to dogs, that 16-pound tabby gave an awful lot of emotional support and brain therapy without asking for much in return.

Reinvented Usefulness

Many people look forward to retirement as if it's one long vacation in a hammock. They're tired after years of work, and their greatest desire is to rest. Others can't wait to fill the calendar with golf games and lunch dates. There's nothing wrong with golf or lunch or hammocks, but let's not take things *too* easy. I have watched several retirees do this, and it never goes well physically, mentally, or in any other way.

Instead, let's find fulfillment by scratching a deeper itch. One of my husband's seminary professors wisely said, "After retirement, there is more life to live and more living in life." He spends his post-teaching years leading seminars, teaching classes, and mentoring younger people with his vast knowledge and loving heart. And without the daily responsibilities of department meetings and a heavy academic schedule, he has more time to freely pursue his God-given passions.

It is inspiring to see the efforts of some of our retired friends who have reinvented themselves when they are no longer collecting a paycheck. One amazing couple who got married in their early eighties combines her vocation as a talented pianist and organist with his gift for singing.

Together they bring joy to many people as they give concerts in churches, nursing homes, and retirement communities. They are busy giving of themselves even though they have to schedule performances around doctor's appointments and physical therapy. As a widow and widower who find comfort in each other, their desire is to share love and encouragement with lonely people who are hurting. They see needs and use their talents to meet them. A sense of usefulness buoys their sense of worth as others are blessed by their music.

Another great guy named Marv was once a high school industrial arts teacher. With summers free, he chose to serve God on many mission trips, from Africa to South America to Alaska. In retirement he had even more time to share his expertise in helping roof buildings and build houses, decks, and ramps. He served with gusto and joy, helping others wherever he could. He did so much work to better the lives of native Alaskans that he was honored by that state for his generous service.

Even as he vacationed in Florida, Marv couldn't sit still by the pool. Instead he grabbed his hammer and tool belt, gathered a few friends, and sought out a local Habitat for Humanity project where workers were needed.

Whether we have arrived at retirement age or not, let's consider what those years may hold. For the sake of this world with its multitude of needs, and for the sake of our own minds and bodies, which thrive on usefulness, let's invest in the places where our passions put fire in the belly.

What will it be for you? Feeding and clothing the poor? Welcoming strangers? Fighting illiteracy? Visiting the sick or imprisoned? Teaching the undernourished to cook? Helping a single parent?

Or perhaps you have put aside artistic interests for a long time. Could it be you've waited until retirement to carve wood or paint? My weaving loom sits like a lonely, neglected friend in our living room, waiting for the day I'll have time to warp and weave. For me it's a symbol of constructive pleasure yet to come. And who knows, perhaps I'll find a young weaver wannabe to share my love of fiber arts.

Pouring ourselves into the next generation is wonderfully rewarding. When I think back to being 25, I remember how my husband and I valued our time with several special couples in their seventies and eighties. They took the time to get to know us. They invited us to dinner, suggested books, taught us how to make pickles, and listened to our young, idealistic thoughts. They didn't judge, though they knew volumes more about life than we did. Today, we still feel the warmth of their friendship and the power of their influence. They gave us more than they ever knew.

Think back over your life. What has been your work? What is your passion? In Ephesians 2:10, Paul speaks of us as "God's handiwork, created in Christ Jesus to do good works, which God prepared in advance for us to do." I believe God puts passion in us to accomplish good things for Him throughout our lives. Our purpose transcends our years on the job.

If the gift of retirement is already your reality, don't just take the golden handshake and retreat. Ask yourself, *How will I leave my mark?* You might not know how valuable your time and attention can be when they are given to others. But knowing isn't what matters. The joy of pouring out blessings on others and feeling useful? That is reward enough for now.

Grateful Heart, Peaceful Mind

Writing thank-you notes was a post-holiday activity that was a blast when our kids were little. It was an art project with a purpose, even if mailing was complicated by children who insisted that only three-dimensional creations could sufficiently express their thanks. Eventually they learned to make pop-up cards. (Thank goodness!)

But those thank-you writing sessions fell from popularity as soon as the kids decided they wanted to share their gratitude without my oversight. I got it, and I changed my tack to gentle reminders: "Do you need any stamps? You do have Papa's address, right?"

Of course, we want our children to have grateful hearts. But what about our own hearts, and what does this mean for our brains? A truly fascinating area of brain research is newly underway at several universities. Scientists are out to understand how gratitude influences what is going on in our head. This, of course, affects how we feel and the way we treat others. At Indiana University, researchers used brain scans to learn how expressing gratitude affected the thought processes of people who were in therapy for depression and anxiety.

Out of a group of 43 clients, 22 spent 20 minutes of 3 therapy sessions writing words of gratitude to a specific recipient. This equaled one hour of expressing thanks. The other 23 people simply attended their regular therapy session. Upon scanning all 43 people at 2 weeks and 3 months afterward, it was easy to see which people expressed gratitude and which ones hadn't. The study continued further, giving the "thankful people" a chance to give away money. Those who expressed the greatest thanks experienced unique activity in the frontal, occipital, and parietal lobes of the brain. The most exciting part of the study is the long-lasting effects that sharing thankfulness seems to have. Participants in the study reported that the more they gave thanks, the more likely they felt grateful. In other words, practicing thankfulness promotes more thankfulness. It bubbles up from our hearts spontaneously.[1]

This has certainly been the case for my friend Jane. A few years ago, Jane and a handful of women read Ann Voskamp's book *One Thousand Gifts*, about a woman who recorded a thousand blessings in her journal. As they read, Jane's group gathered twice a month to discuss the book. Because of that experience, Jane felt moved to write down blessings, large and small, that she noticed each day. Unlike Ann, she doesn't carry a notebook around to record the truly wonderful things as they happen. Instead, Jane makes her bullet-point list each morning as she reviews the previous day.

In her own relaxed manner, Jane doesn't date her entries or stress over how they are written. She just gives each one a number and moves on. The results have been nothing short of amazing, as her list, at the time of this writing, stands at 7,325 blessings! At first Jane felt thankful for special things—old friends who stopped by unexpectedly or a visit to see her grandsons. But as time passed, Jane began thanking God for whatever *is*.

Now she looks for God in the mundane of every day. Upon waking in the night, instead of feeling frustrated that sleep is lost, she thanks God for time with Him and prays for whomever He brings to mind. She is grateful for a mother and baby deer eating from her apple tree, or a loon call that breaks the morning silence over the lake. And out of each experience of true thankfulness, Jane sees God show up more and more. Like the laughing loon, God pierces through the mundane. He is in the everyday. Every day.

The fact that Jane's gratitude list is so long is truly beautiful, especially considering that she lost her beloved husband, unexpectedly, several years ago. She works deeply through the pain of missing Chuck, though she didn't start writing her thanks because of grief. She has noticed, however, that being aware and thanking God encourages her to lift her head in the midst of sadness to sense God's presence. Jane is not one to slap a Band-Aid on a bleeding wound. She is realistic about heartache. She faces it head on. But she is also extremely thankful, and she notices the good things, one by one. Above her work desk hangs a piece of art that says, "*Eucharisteo.*" Or, "Give thanks!"

Jane also realized, as did those researchers who study the effects of gratitude, that being grateful is contagious. As we are thankful people, we are more likely to reach out to others in a positive way. When Jane shares something that causes her to pause and give thanks, joy and gratitude spill over to those around her. This is no surprise. Grateful words are encouraging words, and who couldn't do with a bit of encouragement? One gratitude study indicates that couples who express thanks for each other have more positive feelings about the relationship. This creates a safe environment in which they can deal with relational concerns.[2]

Developing a heart of thankfulness may take effort at first. But, as Jane discovered, it is a self-perpetuating practice. A drop of awareness and thanks becomes a flowing stream of gratitude. Let's be swept up in a current of gratitude that washes over us and makes positive changes in our brains.

One study reports that thankful people also have a greater sense of optimism. They feel more like exercising, and they require fewer visits to the doctor.[3] In the Bible, Paul writes that we are to "give thanks in all circumstances" (1 Thessalonians 5:18). I imagine he knew that giving thanks was a good thing, but I wonder if he knew just *how* good it is.

WAYS TO EXPRESS YOUR THANKS

- Write a note of thanks to someone who has inspired you. Let him or her know, specifically, what you appreciate.

- Make a phone call to thank someone for what he or she has done for you.

- Beginning today, list five things each day for which you are truly grateful. Perhaps this will become your gratitude journal.

- Right now, take three deep cleansing breaths and thank God for at least three blessings that come to mind.

Relationships of the Grandest Kind

People tend to completely lose their minds when they have a baby, and becoming a grandparent invites an even greater level of insanity. Well, not real insanity...but really, *really* intense love. We have a friend who unapologetically claims that although he thought he loved his two children with his whole heart, it wasn't until he became a grandfather that he began to understand what loving with a whole heart means. His newborn grandson moved in and occupied a place in this man's heart he didn't know existed. Such overwhelming affection was foreign to him until that baby was born.

So it is...God in His wisdom put us into families, steeped richly in layers of generations for good reason. Somehow grandparents are wired with a special unconditional love for grandchildren, and grandchildren for grandparents. The "grand" relationship comes especially equipped with extra measures of grace, forgiveness, and love that are sometimes not as easily grasped in the parent-child relationship. Did God know that we needed the aged among us to love little ones in a special way? Does it take a few more decades of living to spawn perspective that lavishes grace? I believe so. And this extraordinary grace is not just passed down from older to younger; it is offered up to the older generation as well. I've seen grandchildren who have unstoppable love for grandparents that skips over middle-aged parents who are caught between trying to balance everyone's needs.

My mother, who was a patient soul, occasionally flashed in frustration while caring for her aging mother. That's when grandchildren could step in with tolerance uncomplicated by tangled strands of the mother-daughter relationship. Grandchildren, who perhaps sensed the deep affection of grandparents when they were little, return that love freely and beautifully, overlooking faults.

And what a gift these relationships are to both the young and the old. Both generations benefit. For children, history comes alive as they hear firsthand experiences of the world their elders knew years ago. Grandparents, who naturally want the best for grandkids, offer wisdom and advice that may be more palatable coming from them than from parents. And kids are helpful to grandparents when they explain ideas of their own generation. There's nothing more interesting than listening to a conversation of substance between a sharp 85-year-old and a millennial. Their perspectives of the world differ, encouraging growth through open, honest communication. Boston College conducted a study showing that a close relationship between grandparents and young adult grandchildren helps both groups experience fewer depressive symptoms, such as sad emotions.[1]

This Christmas as we gathered the family, my 89-year-old dad had 7 of his grandchildren around him. It was a joy to watch him take each one individually and care for them in his special "Papa way." That meant he pulled out his laptop and gave each one a mini-lesson on investing. He talked to them about saving money and investing wisely. He reminded them that hard work is worthwhile and that he came from humble beginnings. What a special thing to watch the way he showed his love for them by imparting bits of his hard-earned wisdom along with lively tales of his youth. We laughed, we cried, we were deeply blessed by the intergenerational abundance of sharing. Naturally there is not complete agreement on all subjects, but respect and love pave the way for valuable conversations.

What a gift for grandchildren to hear from the people who want the best for them no matter what. Grandparents can be the steadiest cheerleaders and the wisest listeners as kids grow up. Often it is grandparents who provide stability if parents break up. They also offer a strong sense of identity, expanding the younger generation's understanding of their place in family history and world history. Our children have heard what it felt like to stand in line at Ellis Island. These are their roots. Their grandparents and great-grandparents were poor immigrants seeking a better life. It is good for them to know, as migration of people is a hot topic in the world today.

For those of us who have or will have grandchildren, let's tell our stories. Let's tell the stories of our parents, grandparents too, as far back as we know. Our history is alive with lessons to be absorbed and appreciated. Such precious tales of the way things worked in 1893 and 1912, 1941 and 1967 hopefully encourage each of us to live better today.

Even if you never have grandchildren, there are plenty of grandparentless children who would benefit from hearing your story. We know a wonderful old retired sea captain whose house is a living history museum complete with steering wheels he rescued off ships that went aground during hurricanes. He warmly welcomes young friends to hear his fascinating tales of life at sea. He also invests in the next generation by praying for twentysomethings to find good spouses as he found when he was 24. The friendship goes both ways, and each end of the relational rope wins.

Mindfulness and the Man with the Yellow Hat

Perhaps you've heard the popular buzzword "mindfulness" and wondered what, exactly, it's all about. To be *mindful* is trendy in psychology and business, as we seek to use our intellects ever more effectively and efficiently. What is it to be mindful? It means different things to different people, but at its base, it means paying *close* attention to whatever is right in front of us. It means silencing the mental noise that blinds us to the present. That sounds simple, but remaining mindful requires effort. For most of us, our thought processes need reforming if we are going to live alert to our surroundings, undistracted by the bombarding din of texts, tweets, and e-mails. Being wide awake to the present experience in which we find ourselves requires effort.

Think of it like this. First thing in the morning, we brush our teeth. Since we do this every morning, we don't have to focus on technique. Our minds are free to wander wherever they feel like going. Within a minute or so, myriad thoughts ricochet in our heads. For me, it's *What will I wear today? Do I have enough time to get my exercises in before work? I want to send so-and-so a birthday card. We need more coffee beans roasted. Is there enough gas in the car, and is the Visa bill paid? Wow, I'm still ticked at the client who gave me a hard time yesterday.*

Glancing in the mirror, I think, *Yikes, I look like my mother today.*

My age is showing. I miss my mom. Too bad she died so young. Oh, I never finished painting the trim in our bathroom. Do I ever finish anything? What shall I start for dinner?

And on and on and on it goes. Meanwhile, I have completely missed the fact that it's snowing beautifully outside the window and six cardinals are taking turns at the feeder. Also, the toothpaste is fresh with mint and the water is clean and cold, which are all lovely gifts.

Remember Curious George, running circles around his ever-patient owner, the man with the yellow hat? George is like that verbose monkey in our heads. He wears us down with his constant chatter. This naughty little guy is persistent, jumping from tree to mental tree, screeching about things we forgot, instances when we performed poorly. Or telling us we're late, unprepared, mad, hurt, or perhaps so worried or sad that we hardly know how to proceed. He makes sure we know we don't measure up in many ways. This confounded animal needs to be silenced. Too bad we can't send him off like Curious George to the care of his benevolent owner, who never seems to grow weary of his pranks. We must form another strategy. What will it be?

First, the nature of the cognitive mind is that it needs to be filled with *something*. So what is it going to be? A yammering chimp who points out all things negative and crushes our souls? In defense of the unruly primate, he might give us a helpful reminder to do something important, such as to pray for that friend who is going through a hard time.

Many things and many people need our attention. It is amazing how many messages fly at us in half a minute: warnings, reminders, discouragement, encouragement, joy, fear, hope, disappointment, shame, longing, anger, disgust, sorrow, frustration, relief, grief, or gratitude. What bubbles to the top? Which items will get the honor of our full attention? That's the question that mindfulness asks each one of us.

Practicing mindfulness means removing the monkey from your shoulder and putting him in a time-out corner. You might thank him for the reminder to send Aunt Susie a birthday card and write that little task on a piece of paper. Maybe you even need to stock your bathroom with three-by-five cards on which to write your to-dos. Then tell George, "I've got this. You can go to your corner and zip it."

The method by which many practice mindfulness is to meditate in the Eastern tradition of sitting quietly and emptying the mind. This is not what I am suggesting. Rather, let's pay attention to our surroundings through the senses that God gave us. As we eat, let us taste. As we walk, let us hear the sounds of the forest, or the neighborhood. And let us look about us and truly see the beauty of creation. That is what I consider meditation.

Some years ago, on a student trip, I realized that the shutter of my camera was stuck, preventing me from capturing the beauty of my surroundings on film. At first I was crushed, but I decided to deeply drink in every scene and smell, knowing I would probably never travel to this part of the world again. To this day, Greece remains etched in my memory: tall Corinthian columns, stone stairways, shimmering Mediterranean waters, roasting lamb, misty mountain roads, and city congestion. With no camera in hand, I was more present than ever to each amazing place and sensation I encountered.

Practicing mindfulness benefits our brains in specific ways. It is not just an idea that somebody invented to increase human productivity. Rather, mindfulness causes positive changes in our brains. Science has shown us how. Mindfulness creates greater effectiveness of the anterior cingulate cortex, the part of the brain that keeps me focused on writing right now rather than running for a desired chunk of chocolate. Impulse control, reward anticipation, and error detection happen in this part of the brain. That's why I can wait until later for a bite of chocolate.

Also, mindfulness increases the density of our gray matter in the prefrontal cortex. This improves decision making, planning, problem solving, and emotion control. And the good old hippocampus, that part of the brain that governs memory and learning, is encouraged to work better as we practice present-moment awareness (meditation). By doing so, we ease stress and decrease depression.[1]

Lastly, the fight-or-flight amygdala of the brain shrinks following meditation. This increases our ability to concentrate.[2] As we have seen, the amygdala is the brain's center for fearful, anxious emotions. With regular meditation, the effects of these energy-zapping emotions diminish.

As we allow ourselves to be present in the precious moments (and the ordinary moments) of life, we nudge our brains toward more healthful function. So let's focus on good things. Let's nourish our minds rather than empty them.

In the next chapter we'll explore the Bible's version of mindfulness: keeping our minds *full* of the goodness that God, in His wisdom, knows we need.

Mind the Good Stuff

As we discussed in the previous chapter, mindfulness does not have to mean emptying the mind, as some Eastern religions prescribe. Rather, as Christians, the waves of our focus flow in the other direction. We need to fill up our minds with the grace, peace, and love of Christ. Realizing that God made us and all that is around us, we honor Him by paying close attention to the present. As C.S. Lewis said in *Letters to Malcom, Chiefly on Prayer*, "The real labor is to attend. In fact, to come awake."

In other words, let's pay attention to life's small wonders rather than flying through our days and straining to accomplish more than is humanly possible.

Yes, our lives are complicated. Sometimes we eat with cell phones on the table, drawing our attention away from the people we dine with. Our racing and triple-tasking stress our minds, especially when we give too much credence to the negative monkey chatter rattling around in our noggins.

But let's change our focus. Let's listen to words from Scripture, words that are polar opposites to negative chimp chat. In Psalm 46:10 we read, "Be still, and know that I am God." This is just one verse that provides a solid framework for Christian meditation.

Here's what Christian meditation can look like. Let's begin by focusing on our breathing. Inhale slowly while saying to yourself, *Be still and know*. Then, as you slowly exhale, think, *that I am God*. Sitting in a comfortable position with shoulders relaxed, repeat this over and over, allowing God's presence to surround and envelop you.

Perhaps you have another favorite verse from the Bible. Slowly breathe in and out, repeating a few comforting words of that verse. Doing this for five to ten minutes each day is an effective form of meditation. In this simple practice, we are more aware of Christ's presence in our heads and our hearts.

Meditation like this helps set the direction for our brains. When we focus our thoughts on good and wholesome things, we are more likely to cultivate feelings of contentment and warmheartedness.[1]

When we fail to focus in positive directions, our untethered brain might wander in the opposite direction, down dark paths of rumination. Rumination comes from Latin *ruminatio* (or *rumen*). The rumen is the first compartment in the digestive system of a cow. It is where the cow's food lands first and meets microbes that begin a fermentation process. Next, the cow regurgitates this mass, which we know as a cud, and gnaws on it some more before swallowing it once again.

So rumination means to chew the cud, or to turn something over and over in the mind. If you are thinking, *Ew...that's gross*, you're right. This behavior is best kept in the bovine world. But we humans ruminate in our brains. We regurgitate, in a sense, the bitter pills we have swallowed, and then we chew on them, allowing that negativity to permeate. We become worrywarts, worn out by all that mental chewing.

Jesus had very specific words for us about worry.

> Do not worry about your life, what you will eat or drink; or about your body, what you will wear. Is not life more than food, and the body more than clothes? Look at the birds of the air; they do not sow or reap or store away in barns, and yet your heavenly Father feeds them. Are you not much more valuable than they? Can any one of you by worrying add a single hour to your life? (Matthew 6:25-27).

I believe our heavenly Father realized our tendency to rehash the painful words, thoughts, and experiences that can send our minds into a negative vortex. Meditating on the goodness of Scripture, spoken in love, encourages our hearts.

As we try to battle worry, it's also helpful to engage our bodies in activities that require our mental attention. For example, we might play the piano or another instrument or sing. When I sing with my choir or play the piano, my mind is unable to chew that negative, emotionally draining cud.

If making music isn't your thing, doing Pilates or dancing ballet both use the body and mind beautifully, encouraging meditative release.

As we fill ourselves with wholesome goodness, we displace the negative, worrisome weight that so easily fills our minds. This is not the same thing as watching a movie. That is simply a distractor. We may put ourselves in the story, but eventually the credits roll, the lights come up, and there we are, squinting at a world that's no better than it was when the theater went dark.

So to deal effectively with worry, let's *intentionally* focus our thoughts on what we are doing. Picture a dancer who counts steps and memorizes choreography. She strives to communicate through the movement of her body and the beauty of the dance. And that process benefits her mind as well as her body.

Here's another Scripture worthy of our meditation. Philippians 4:8-9 expresses perfectly what we are to put into our heads, which thoughts we need to focus on when we feel the darkness of the world closing in. Read these words slowly, taking in the meaning of each one.

> Finally brothers and sisters, whatever is true, whatever is noble, whatever is right, whatever is pure, whatever is lovely, whatever is admirable—if anything is excellent or praiseworthy—think about such things. Whatever you have learned or received or heard from me—put it into practice. And the God of peace will be with you.

As we choose to live with our minds focused on what we are doing—looking expectantly for God to show up in the present moment—we attach our deepest selves to Christ. Our minds are renewed and our spirits strengthened. Filling ourselves with Christ is to enjoy the best brain food ever.

Faith Is Forever

I am the first to admit that Alzheimer's disease is one of the worst illnesses ever known to humankind. The way it sneaks in and steals a person's identity is nothing short of criminal. While it is disorienting for the person with the disease, it's also incredibly unsettling to watch a loved one descend into the murky darkness that disguises him or her almost beyond recognition.

Often, people suffering from this disease can no longer enjoy their favorite books, songs, hobbies, and everyday routines. Quality of life is ravaged.

My dear father-in-law, Paul, has been suffering with Alzheimer's for the past nine years. It is a progressive illness, meaning it gets worse and worse, never better. It's torture to see his once-sharp cognition and memory drain away bit by bit. One month he understands what to do with a fork and a handkerchief; the next they are worthless objects. Not long ago he still knew his spouse, children, and grandchildren. Today he remembers only his most consistent loved one—his caring wife of 60 years.

On many levels, the process is painful for each of us. We still see Paul's endearing mannerisms and handsome face. His lovely eyes are still brilliant blue, but much of the time their sparkle has been replaced by a vacant look. Once in a while, we catch a glimmer of recognition and joy, but those are rare moments coaxed by a piece of chocolate or a grandchild who encourages Paul to wiggle his ears (one of his best tricks).

My pet theory is that even though Paul can't say or do what he used to, vital thoughts are still going on in his head. Beliefs still remain in his heart. These paramount bits of knowledge and truth have stuck with him longer than anything else. His sister, Susie, is able to talk him through childhood memories that elicit hearty guffaws. She takes Paul on mental tours of their old neighborhood, tours still cataloged in a part of his brain that is intact. New memories are fleeting, but Paul's recollection of the pale yellow foursquare house on Charles Street in Jamestown, New York, is crystal clear. He responds with animated looks of happiness and laughs at all the right places when Susie describes the antics of their youth.

Best of all, Paul has not forgotten Jesus.

A retired pastor, he smiles when his caregivers call him Pastor Paul. And when almost nothing in his world makes any sense, he still knows what it means to pray and read the Bible. Sometimes when I visit, I ask, "Paul, would you like me to read from the book of Psalms or from the book of John?" I'm just testing him. I know John is his favorite. He frequently preached from John's gospel during his years as a pastor. So far, his answer hasn't surprised me. "John!" he says emphatically. As I read to him, he closes his eyes and listens intently. He is drinking in words that are like old friends to him, old friends of the dearest kind.

When I finish, his eyes open, and he nods approvingly. Sometimes he even says, "Good!"

Paul's faith is bedrock. For him, the love of Christ, so clearly spelled out in the book of John, is deeply engraved on the walls of his soul. When so little else is comprehensible, his faith remains.

Of course, we don't know *exactly* what is happening in Paul's brain because his words are mostly unintelligible, but we do know that the most important aspect of his life remains solid. And how incredible it is that the essence of Paul Sparrman, like all of us mortals, is wrapped up in the personhood of God? Could it be that Paul is in a no-man's-land, an in-between place? Perhaps one foot is on earth and the other is in heaven. I certainly don't have the answer, but I think it's evident that in Paul's earlier, comprehending life, he built a foundation of faith that is carrying him on to eternal life with his Savior.

Even in the midst of Paul's Alzheimer's, we are treated to beautiful sightings of God's grace shining through one of his followers. I don't wish to romanticize the suffering that comes with Alzheimer's. But we cannot ignore the surprising glimpses of joyful faith that flash bright against the inky darkness of dementia. Paul, despite his confusion, still loves Jesus. I believe he will always keep this knowledge close to his heart. And when his earthly days are exchanged for heavenly ones, he will be free from the shackles of Alzheimer's. His faith, which now is very childlike, will expand to a new fullness in the presence of Christ. At least that's how I see it.

Meanwhile, we will live with hope in what seems like a hopeless situation. And we will follow Paul's example of building a solid faith in Jesus, a faith that will go the distance.

Do Not Be Afraid

It's not every day that we are invited to the ninety-fifth birthday of a friend who is so incredibly with-it and wise. But such was a party we recently attended. Helen, seated at the center of the table, showed her usual warm countenance. She was surrounded by nine friends and family members who felt honored to celebrate this remarkable woman.

It was fascinating to learn more of Helen's younger years as the daughter of Armenian immigrants who came to the United States during the aftermath of the Armenian Genocide of 1915 to 1917. Her family left Turkey under terrifying circumstances, even losing a couple of Helen's older siblings in their narrow escape.

One might guess that such devastating violence would taint the family tree with a spirit of bitterness. But thanks to the bedrock faith of her mother, Helen grew up knowing God's love and peace. Her family settled in rural Pennsylvania. Her mom, grateful to just be alive, looked forward to their new life rather than looking back at all they lost.

When Helen was just 19, she moved to Washington, DC, to work in the office of the surgeon general. It was her job to assign new physicians, fresh out of medical school, to their places of service as World War II heated up. She wisely declined bribes from desperate fathers who called to influence the placement of their sons. They promised her fancy trips to New York City as well as nylon stockings (which were high-ticket items during the war). It took a lot of courage to suddenly become a city girl with a challenging job. Living in Washington was a far cry from home in the bucolic Pennsylvania countryside.

Helen remembers a night when she was filled with a sense of awe as she looked up at the illuminated dome of the Capitol building. Excitement thrilled her heart, but she also felt a twinge of fear. When asked what advice the Helen of today would give to her teenaged self, she firmly answers, "Do not be afraid!"

Fear was a demon to be wrested to the ground. How could one not feel frightened when war raged and uncertainty lay heavily over the world? As a girl whose family experienced devastating consequences of war, Helen sometimes felt that fear might crush her soul beyond repair. But Helen experienced God's companionship and provision all her life. She watched her mother, who clung to God through the loss of loved ones, home, and homeland. Such tragedy could have consumed her. But divine intervention offers calm. It produces the kind of indescribable peace that we see in Helen today. She is calm balm, generously giving herself to others.

In return, she is blessed with rich relationships, a peaceful heart, and clarity of mind.

We love Helen's indomitable spirit and the way she connects so well with others. Her intense interest in people's lives is testament to her selfless attitude. With genuine enthusiasm, she asks about all the children of the guests at her birthday dinner. She listens intently. When my husband inquires about her secret for being so young at 95, she says with a laugh, "I feel young because all my friends are young."

Of course, 95-year-olds don't have many peers, but the ninetysomethings who befriend younger people understand the great value of giving and receiving in relationships.

The Helen who left the country for a big-city job at 19, the Helen who moved to Cyprus for her husband's work in 1959, and the one who raised three daughters and a son are all evident in the Helen of today. When I look at her thoughtful face and try to imagine all the living she has done for nine and a half decades, I see beauty and grace in her gentle eyes. Those eyes clearly reflect love and a strong faith in Jesus Christ.

Helen gets up each day with a pragmatic spirit. She does what needs to be done. Two of her daughters happen to live overseas—one in Paris and the other in London. She has grandchildren whose home is in Portugal. They lead busy lives and come to the US to see her when they are able, but most of their visits happen in Europe. Helen is accustomed to boarding transatlantic flights to be with her family. She flies across oceans as nonchalantly as others might catch the Metro downtown.

Without fanfare or any thought that people in their nineties might find long-distance travel a burden, Helen simply states that if she wants to remain in the lives of her family, she must go. Besides, she thinks sitting on a plane for eight or nine hours is no big deal.

This commitment to travel epitomizes Helen's desire to stay engaged in the lives of friends and family. These valuable relationships also keep her vitally connected to the world and all its changes and challenges. Living in her son and daughter-in-law's home allows her the side benefit of knowing two grandsons very well. They are fortunate boys to grow up experiencing Helen's wisdom every day. She loves it when they come down to her apartment to play a game or troubleshoot her computer.

Technology is an important tool for her. It allows her to stay close to those she loves. Her zest for life and her outward focus are a bright light for others. As she opens her arms to people around her, she is embraced by many friends, friends who are more than happy to share her vitality and joy. Helen inspires us to choose faith in Christ, even when life is hard. She has clearly taken her own advice to live without fear. And she thrives in relationships that outshine any dullness that might accompany those who live in isolation.

Whether we are 19 or 90, let's not underestimate the paramount importance of spiritual and relational vitality. Closeness with our heavenly Father and attention to relationships with other people promote the vivacious spirit that Helen's life exemplifies.

54

Choosing to Be Brave

I feel ill-equipped to say anything about bravery, but this subject seems tied to keeping our minds sharp. Sounds crazy perhaps, but hear me out.

During my years as an RN, I cared for many people in their homes. Being a home-health nurse gave me a peek into many delightful elderly people's personal lives. Some patients and their families warmly welcomed me, a young and inexperienced nurse who was sometimes their only contact with the outside world.

Others were a little more suspicious, thinking that maybe I was a high school student posing as their nurse of the day. Eventually most folks learned to trust me as I changed dressings, drew blood, reviewed medications and diets, and did my best to encourage healing and health.

Over time, I discovered that I could divide my patients into two categories. There were the brave ones and the not-so-brave ones, the "Braves" and the "Wimpies." (Of course, I couldn't write those words in my charting notes.)

The Braves pushed themselves hard, even when pain flared, wounds didn't want to close, or chemotherapy made eating an awful chore. On that one day of the week when they were not halted by nerve pain, they went out for walks. They smiled at simple pleasures, like sunshine across a quilt-covered bed or the smell of coffee. They didn't complain when I said I had to draw blood or put them through the uncomfortable indignity of changing a catheter. They asked questions about me and listened for my answers. Such brave souls they were, beautiful and inspiring, each in his or her own way.

Then there were the Wimpies. I should say right away that they all get a pass because they suffered from pain, poverty, or both. Hope had been squeezed from them a long time ago. Still, they were the hard visits, which I tried to sandwich in between the less taxing ones. Sometimes their living conditions flagged to depressing levels. If I had to exist in some of the apartments I visited, I would be sad and worried too. And depressed.

Combine illness with really crummy surroundings, and disease prevails. There were old men dying of lung cancer who couldn't stop smoking clouds of foul air that their families also had to breathe. A couple of people were hostile to me, assuming I was a spoiled girl come to criticize their hard luck. Occasionally I encountered illegal drugs. Once I was bitten by a pit bull who sensed his owner's hostility toward me.

But tough circumstances aside, there was still a divide between those who chose bravery and those who found the need to focus on all that was bad.

It wasn't the living situation or medical diagnosis that determined a patient's outlook. Some of my dearest old people were fearless in the worst of circumstances. They were brave in body and spirit. They pushed themselves to do the best they could against rotten odds. They didn't give up easily, physically or mentally. An obstacle that might cause one person to give up was just another hill for these intrepid folks to climb.

One of my patients was like young Margaret Dashwood in Jane Austen's *Sense and Sensibility.* At one point in the story, the perfectly healthy Margaret whimpers, "I'm not *supposed* to run!" That attitude of "sit still and protect the body from sweating" actually does us a disservice. We need to push, stretch, and strive a little harder. This might mean an extra ten minutes on the elliptical machine or an extra dozen laps in the pool. This uptick in effort is different for each person.

But the mind-set that encourages a harder run toward physical health or brain health is the same.[1] Am I going to live like my brave patients whose mental determination allowed them to reach admirable goals? Or will I be a Wimpie who chooses to remain sedentary, with my legs elevated weeks after the doctor has given me the green light to start walking?

Challenging our bodies and brains keeps them strong and functional. Let us be brave in our physical activity, and let's continue to bravely flex our brains every way we can.

Brave Thinking

In the previous chapter, I mentioned my brave patients who exerted themselves physically. Now let's focus on the mental aspect of exertion. And take heart—I'm not saying we have to start doing brain-straining calculus problems.

Instead, I want to encourage telling the truth inside our own heads. We don't intend to deceive ourselves, but it is easy to stuff feelings and obfuscate the truth when facing that truth is painful and stressful. This practice of inwardly denying negative feelings can become habit forming. This causes problems for our brains. If we aren't able to consciously admit to ourselves what is gnawing away at our psyches, we are unable to deal healthfully with the concerns that plague the depths of our souls.

I'm not suggesting that we dump our emotions on a gut-spilling Facebook post, or wear our hearts on our sleeves. But we need to be able to name our deep struggles and difficult emotions. We need to confront those inner struggles so they won't sabotage us or even drain the life out of us.

Life is not all neat and tidy and happy. Optimism is great. If we can see the cup as half full rather than half empty, how wonderful! But let's be realistic; life brings struggles, disappointments, and pain. That is just an unavoidable fact.

What's up for grabs, however, is how we choose to deal with the hardships and heartaches that come our way. Will we deal with them honestly? Or will they be buried deep inside, where they can insidiously wreak havoc in our lives?

For many summers, we hosted a houseguest who worked a seemingly impossible job. She was often in the public eye—and loved by many people. But she also received more than her fair share of criticism and blame. On the surface, she appeared to take it all in stride. She batted away all of the personal attacks as if they were pesky flies. When vacation hit, however, she was inevitably stretched out in our family room with her feet up and a bag of frozen peas draped across her forehead to ease her "end-of-semester migraine." (When she came to visit, we knew we had to keep plenty of icy peas on hand.)

When she spoke of her job, she carefully navigated around the landmines of frustration and worry. She put a positive spin on the challenges, but we could see through the thin veneer of her carefully crafted words. Meanwhile her head pounded with pain. I am not a psychologist, but it didn't require one to see that denial was her coping mechanism of choice. She chose to deny how much it hurt her when her decisions drew sharp criticism.

I remember thinking, *If she could admit, even to herself, that public opinion really does matter to her, it might relieve the power that worry and frustration hold over her.*

Stress, sadness, and pain in our lives are inevitable. It's how we choose to handle these emotional enemies that matters. When we push the negative feelings out of sight and into our subconscious, we prevent our minds from dealing with the mental and emotional baggage that weighs us down. This doesn't do our brains or our bodies any favors. Some people consume bottles of antacids to cope. Others live on ibuprofen or too many martinis after work. But what is really happening? We are denying reality.

It might surprise you to learn that a certain degree of denial can actually be helpful. For example, when we face a horrendous catastrophe, our brains protect us by processing only as much as we can handle in that moment. Then, as we are able to face it, truth is ushered in bit by bit in manageable portions. This is the mental form of shock—denial functioning at its best.

Conversely, denial at its worst happens when our brains trap stress, anxiety, fear, or sadness deep in our subconscious or unconscious minds. In the case of our houseguest, the horror of being criticized rattled around inside of her. As a result, she was stressed out, exhausted, and immobilized by migraine headaches. She thought she should be able to handle all the public (but very personal) attacks on her own. But she couldn't. Her failure to acknowledge this truth allowed her stress to overpower her. This kind of wear and tear on the brain is costly.

When our brains face the pressure of unresolved stress, we suffer from high levels of the glucocorticoid hormones adrenaline, noradrenaline, and cortisol.

When this happens for long periods of time, we enter a state called *cortisol dominance*. This negatively affects concentration, learning, and memory. This is why identifying negative feelings is a valuable step toward brain health. For me, journaling uncovers what is chewing me up inside. For others, talking or praying with a trusted friend or counselor is a helpful way to deal with adversity.

Facing the truth, that "monster in the basement," is the first step to coping. Only after we courageously name our pain, disappointment, or causes of stress—and begin to understand their sources—can we make strides toward emotional healing. By doing so, we also encourage physical health and a brain that functions at its intellectual best. Then, hopefully, we won't need all those frozen peas after all.

Free to Forgive, Forgive to Be Free

Holding on to anger is like allowing a noose to be tied around your neck. Few things are as debilitating as anger. We all know how it feels to be offended, betrayed, and hurt. Sometimes the hurt is unintentional, but sometimes we are hurt with intent.

Whatever the case, pain is as inevitable as the sun rising tomorrow. We are excluded, insulted, lied to, misunderstood, forgotten, cheated on, or perhaps even threatened physically. Many of us are the victims of abuse.

Who hasn't been the butt of a cruel joke or the scapegoat for another's anger? I am sorry to bring up bad memories, but this is real life that we are talking about.

And we must admit that as imperfect humans, we too are guilty of inflicting deep pain on others. How are we to cope with such hard truths? How do we deal with it when we feel trampled by others—when we've been so violated that it feels like our souls are in tatters?

You might be wondering what all of this has to do with the well-being of our brains. It's more than we might realize.

For example, our ability to forgive others benefits us physically, spiritually, and mentally.[1] Clinging to an offense or a relational injury is like falling into water wearing heavy clothes. We struggle, kick, and thrash in a prison of wet garments, all the while exhausting ourselves and sinking deeper.

Getting mad saps our "on-demand" energy. *Staying* mad, however, drains our reserves of energy. Worse yet, it steals our joy. Have you ever relived an offense or betrayal and realized that your heart was pounding and your face felt hot? You're just as upset as when the pain was fresh.

The old anger and hurt still haunt you, looming large and causing emotional waves to crash over your head. *Again and again!*

That's why it's important to create a strategy for returning to the welcoming shores of emotional equilibrium. And if forgiveness is missing from our action plans, turbulence will simmer under the surface. Insidiously, it will damage our inner peace and our relationships with others.

Of course forgiveness is often not our first response when we've been unfairly mistreated. But it's well worth the effort to release our offenders from that penalty box in our heads.

Several university studies have explored what happens in our minds and bodies when we fail to forgive. If we hold on to resentment, mentally reliving a stressful or hurtful situation, our bodies experience a racing pulse, elevated blood pressure, and shallow breathing. We sweat profusely. These physical symptoms negatively affect our brains.[2] When we are angry, we are more likely to experience anxiety and depression, two symptoms that tend to pull us away from relationships and into an isolative state.

Participants in one study reported that holding a grudge makes life seem meaningless.[3] For some, the struggle runs especially deep because it contradicts their spiritual belief that we ought to forgive. So they feel guilt along with their resentment, adding even more weight to an already heavy load.

On the other hand, people who can forgive hurtful offenses most likely enjoy healthier relationships and a stronger sense of self. Research shows that the person who forgives benefits *even more* than the one who is forgiven.[4] Releasing ourselves from the bonds of anger is incredibly freeing. It's important to note here that choosing to forgive doesn't mean we think that mistreatment is acceptable. Abuse, for example, whether either emotional or physical, is never okay. And it certainly was not okay for innocent Amish schoolgirls to be mercilessly shot by an intruder on a normal school day in their peaceful Pennsylvania schoolhouse in 2006. But somehow the families of these victims joined together and moved beyond their unimaginable pain to forgive the killer, even though he was already dead.

The Amish community reached out to the killer's family with support and unconditional love, shocking people across the country. The healing this community experienced is truly remarkable. It is hard to understand how the families of the slain continue to live with a spirit of forgiveness in the absence of the children they love. Not only were innocent lives snuffed out, but so was innocence of this close-knit community.[5]

We must keep in mind that forgiveness is a process. It is nearly impossible to simply decide, *Yes, I will forgive the murderer, the rapist, or the family member who continually causes us grief.* Forgiveness is a journey that takes time. It requires forgiving over and over again as we deal with the ongoing fallout of an offense or injury. It is a struggle that happens deep in our soul. And as crazy as it sounds, the most effective step toward forgiveness is trying to identify with the position of the person who has hurt us. Attempting to walk in his or her shoes for a moment, instead of marinating in bitterness or obsessing about revenge, moves us along the road to forgiveness, a road that leads to freedom.[6]

There is plenty of non-faith-based evidence supporting the fact that forgiveness promotes mental health.[7] But those who know Christ's love have the greatest example of forgiveness. While in desperate agony and close to death, Jesus managed to eke out the words, "Father, forgive them, for they do not know what they are doing" (Luke 23:34). He did the unimaginable. He identified with the feelings of His abusers. He knew they were not equipped to fully grasp their sinfulness.

With Jesus as our example, may we eventually learn to forgive. Disentangling ourselves from resentment and releasing our grudges and anger will bring us the reward of fresh winds of freedom, winds that will refresh our souls. We calm down and breathe easier. This allows our brains to function better.[8]

Choosing empathy and compassion for the one who wronged us is one of the world's greatest stress reducers. This empathy and compassion come from the realization that we all sin.

Not one of us is perfect. We have all hurt somebody at some time or another. When we are able to put ourselves in the other person's shoes, empathy is born and the process of forgiveness may begin.

Conversations with God

It's a humbling experience to visit with a friend who is busily planning her hundredth birthday party. When I sit with Harriet in her lovely home, I can't help notice that her nails, like her house, are perfect, and her hair is better coiffed than mine. The teacups are beautiful, and Harriet holds hers with grace even though she is recovering from a bout of pneumonia. We talk about her full life, which is part history lesson and part primer on modern business and how to effectively train and encourage a sales team. That's because Harriet still works at age 99. I know; she's incredible!

As Harriet shares her recent experience of speaking at a conference, her enthusiasm spills over to other areas of her life. I ask about her professional successes, and we talk about the pain of losing her 36-year-old mother (ironically, to pneumonia) when Harriet was just 12. On top of that, her mom died within months of the 1929 stock market crash, which threatened the livelihood of most Americans.

Harriet doesn't deny that her mother's death was a devastating blow. But so was losing her dad's grocery store during the Great Depression. Harriet is utterly honest about the horror of those days. As was tradition in back in 1929, she and her brothers had to sit on chairs in their living room, next to their mom's casket, while neighbors and friends filed by. "It was *awful*!" she says.

During the young adolescent years that followed, Harriet was poor and heartbroken, suddenly the only female in the home. Each day she came home from school to cook dinner from meager rations for her father and two brothers.

But Harriet's candor about the agony of her youth is equaled by her excitement for life today. What's most amazing is her enthusiasm about the ongoing conversation she has each morning with God. She waves a hand toward the ceiling and tells me how she visits with Jesus every day, reviewing all that happened the day before. She pours out all her concerns to Him: friends who need prayer, family members who wait for healing, and problems that need to be solved.

Harriet talks to God the same way she speaks to me—honestly, thoughtfully, and with complete trust. She knows she is heard. Her daily out-loud conversations with God guide her decision making. She has been communing with God like this for so many years that she can't imagine a morning without it. She tells me, "I wouldn't have survived all these years without my daily heart-to-heart with Jesus. It's the only way I know how to live. It's how I decide what to do next."

Prayer has been Harriet's lifeline for nearly a century. She has faced hardship with such bravery. She lost her mom at 12, and her husband in his midfifties. Yet she harbors no bitterness, and that's because of God's grace in her life. Through candid dialogue, she brings it all to Jesus. She reads the Bible, but other than that she has no specific formula for prayer. She simply talks to God as a trusted friend.

Harriet makes prayer sound so simple. But isn't that what it's supposed to be?

Dr. Andrew Newberg, a renowned researcher in neurology and spirituality at the Thomas Jefferson Hospital and University in Philadelphia, studies the effects of prayer and meditation on the brain. I think he would be delighted to meet Harriet. He would agree that her active prayer life is one reason she is so vibrant and sharp at almost 100. While scanning the brains of people who are deep in prayer, Dr. Newberg observes how the brain is hardwired for faith. Positive physical changes happen in our brains when we pray. This results in decreased stress and a greater ability to react with patience toward others. Also,

Newberg reports that the more we participate in prayer or Bible study, the more our mind wants to do it.[1]

I've heard some people say that believing in God and needing to pray are crutches. They imply that only weak or injured people should use such appliances. Perhaps this is so, but who among us *isn't* weak or injured in some way? Perhaps this is why God, who created our brains, endowed us with a profound need to communicate with Him.

Science affirms that praying promotes better brain function. Dr. Newberg believes that a positive perception of God calms our mind. Conversely, negative thoughts about God increase our internal stress and anxiety. In some cases, this leads to depression.

Dr. Newberg, when asked what he does to keep his brain sharp, produced a list that could have been written by Harriet. First, he gets plenty of cardiovascular exercise and he eats well. He strives to avoid processed foods; fruits and veggies dominate his diet. He believes that by encouraging a healthy physical body, his spiritual life is enhanced. In other words, he concurs with the apostle Paul, who likens our bodies to temples of the Holy Spirit (1 Corinthians 6:19). Dr. Newberg champions continued learning, whether by taking a class, staying current with world affairs, or attending a play.

Further, due to his understanding of what happens in the brain during prayer, he encourages us to keep the faith and practice spiritual disciplines. He says that "faith, in the broadest sense, is the best thing you can have for the brain."[2]

Combining Dr. Newberg's science with what we learn from faithful people like Harriet, I feel doubly encouraged about the importance of frequent conversations with God. I agree with Harriet and with many others who live by this quote: "I don't know what the future holds—but I know who holds the future." Amen! Let us pray.

Drinking from the Half-Full Cup

Are you a "cup half full" or "cup half empty" person? This question is the classic indicator of whether a person sees himself or herself as an optimist, trying to look on the bright side, or a pessimist, wallowing in negative thoughts and often blaming oneself.

For example, if one of our kids breaks out in poison ivy rashes on the first day at the beach, do we instantly assume the entire vacation is ruined?

On the other hand, if someone in the house wakes up early to brew coffee and make pancakes, does it set our heart racing with a joy that catapults us out of bed with happy gusto?

Did you know that when we allow positive thoughts to dominate our brains' neural pathways, a cascade effect triggers even more favorable thoughts? This gives the brain a boost that helps it function more effectively.

Woo-hoo! Keeping in mind that brain plasticity means our brains are constantly changing, let's consider the way optimistic people think. These folks acknowledge that life is not easy. It is filled with challenges that can break our hearts and wear us down.

Yet optimists face challenges in a way that is realistic yet hopeful. They see the difficulties but are not annihilated by their force. In looking for the best possible outcome in a situation, their brains search for positive solutions. Optimists are generally cheerful and live longer. They creatively handle life's inevitable difficulties.[1]

The psychological makeup of a positive person promotes greater physical well-being, including less cardiovascular disease and even better protection from the common cold.[2]

But what if I am a naturally pessimistic person (or as many pessimists contend, a *realist*)? Well, thank goodness for brain plasticity because it offers hope for the Eeyores among us. It is possible to retrain the brain to choose more positive ways of processing the world.

Let's start attending to our own self-talk, that stream of consciousness that fills our minds with chatter when our brains are free to wander. It's valuable to listen to this self-talk. As we walk to the car with a bag of groceries or run a letter to the mailbox, what kinds of conversations are going on in our heads?

It's helpful to stop ourselves in midthought several times a day and ask, *Which mental road am I taking? Am I condemning someone? Or am I grateful for the friend whose letter I can't wait to answer? Do I notice crocuses popping bravely through the snow? Or am I grumbling that the snow is dirty and I'm sick of winter?*

If a person or circumstance causes us to anxiously ruminate, it's wise to check our thoughts. Psychologist Dr. Linda Solie, author of *Take Charge of Your Emotions,* helps us look objectively at the cause of our stress. In her book, she offers several tools for dealing effectively with anxiety. In one method, she recommends writing down the stressful issue and peeling back each layer of the problem one by one and noting, "...which is a problem because..." at each level. For example:

I am terrified to try out for college choir, even though I want to be in it.

- Which is a problem because I might sing badly and not make it.

- Which is a problem because all my friends will make it.

- Which is a problem because I'll feel envious of those who are selected.

- Which is a problem because I will feel humiliated and left out.

- Which is a problem because my pride will feel injured and I will feel sad.

- Which is a problem because it reinforces the idea that I am not good at anything, and I'm a worthless person.

- Which is a problem because worthless people have nothing to offer.

- Which is a problem because with nothing to offer at college, I might as well quit and go home.

- Which is a problem because I would rather die than do that!

And, *ah-ha*! I have finally landed in the basement of my negative thinking, thinking that prevented me from auditioning for something I really want. Each of those "which is a problem" scenarios was a step to arriving at the core issue: I don't feel very good about myself right now. Finally, while crouching in the basement of my thoughts, I'm able to laugh at myself and realistically ask, "Am I really such a worthless individual?"

From this place I can see that my negative thinking is ridiculous and unproductive. I may not have what it takes to sing in college choir, but surely other opportunities are available. Turning our minds to more positive thought processes applies to many areas of our lives, including thoughts about our own brain health.[3]

The fact that you are reading this book tells me that keeping your mind sharp is important to you. Fantastic! How about engaging optimistic thoughts about that goal? It is natural for each of us to experience little memory lapses. This is part of life. I'm encouraged to remember how many times I misplaced keys or even a passport in my early twenties. And we know it's normal to have more "senior moments" as we age. But let's take these things for what they are—typical annoyances. Let's not assume the worst. My husband, whose father has been all but consumed by Alzheimer's (and whose sweet mother has advanced dementia) refuses to believe that his parents' mental declines write the ticket for him.

If he succumbed to a self-fulfilling prophecy, I would be worried. Instead, disciplined, regular exercise and good nutrition are keeping his body in shape. Plus, plenty of music and intellectual stimulation feed his mind and soul. He is what I call a realistic optimist.

None of us can clearly predict the future. We can't guess which parts of us will wear out first, but attempting to deal honestly with stress promotes positive thinking—and positive thinking encourages brain health. Last evening, my husband and I shared supper with a retired psychiatrist and his wife. With a twinkle in his eye, the good doctor agreed that optimism serves the brain more effectively than most drugs. This nearly 90-year-old couple's buoyant spirits are living proof that there's truth in the "positive pudding."

Whose Body Is It?

For a moment, let's consider our bodies, brains included, from the perspective of the One who made us. King David wrote in Psalm 139:13-14, "You created my inmost being; you knit me together in my mother's womb. I praise you because I am fearfully and wonderfully made; your works are wonderful, I know that full well."

In His holy wisdom, God dreamed up humankind, and here we are, living souls inhabiting living bodies. Each day our minds make many choices that affect our bodies. And what happens with our bodies, in turn, affects our cognitive capacity. As the culmination of God's creation, we humans are made in His image. Certainly, then, our heavenly Father cares about the way we treat ourselves in mind, body, and spirit.

Scripture has plenty to say about the Holy Spirit, who inhabits our bodies. First Corinthians 6:19-20 says, "Do you not know that your bodies are temples for the Holy Spirit, who is in you, whom you have received from God? You are not your own; you were bought at a price. Therefore honor God with your bodies."

We wouldn't think of making a new batch of yogurt in a jar that wasn't perfectly clean. In making good yogurt, the container matters. Why would we allow our body to be polluted? It's the vessel that holds our true self—our spirit. Some say, "The body is just a shell." That might be true, but this is the only shell we get for our lives on earth.

So shouldn't we take good care of the body God gave us? Shouldn't we consider our bodies in this light?

Other people take another view. "It's my body," they say. "I can do with it what I wish." But is it really yours *exclusively*? Doesn't God, the Artist who created us, have a say in what happens to what He made?

As a believer in Jesus Christ, I'm certain of one thing: Jesus loves me. Not only that, but despite my moments of doubts and questions, I believe He loved me enough to die for me. This is great news because I am sinful, and only His sacrifice can make me clean.

If this is sounds like a crazy, radical idea to you, I encourage you to grab a Bible and read the Gospel of John. John spells things out clearly in John 3:16. God loves humankind so much that He allowed His Son, Jesus, to die so that when we die, we'll be raised to new life—a perfect life with Him. Meanwhile, however, our souls, the essence of who we are, are contained in the bodies we were born with. Therefore, the way we choose to care for our bodies *matters*.

Sometimes we might feel this is a losing battle, especially as our bodies degrade through the natural process of aging. Sure, our knees get crackly, and wrinkles are inevitable. But honestly, I don't think aging is the worst thing that happens to us.

It's all the other deleterious things we do to our bodies that harm them most. We often overeat and overdrink. Or we eat the wrong things and take no notice of the difference between calories consumed and calories burned. At times we might ignore our need for good exercise. Not to beat a dead horse, but what happens in our bodies below the neck influences what goes on above our necks, namely in our brains.

And what about the emotions we harbor—love, hate, envy? Are we capable of compassion, or are we more concerned with getting even? We have talked about what happens to our container when we run wild with anger, refuse to forgive, and hold tightly to stress. Loads of research states that the condition of the soul plays a major role in our ability to think.

While this book may seem *too* chock-full of ways to keep your brain functioning at full tilt, if you are feeling overwhelmed, please relax.

Perhaps it hasn't been your habit to swim, hike, breathe deeply, journal, write letters, eat loads of vegetables, make yogurt, learn a new language, tend a garden, join a book group, or make music. So trying to implement all these changes immediately seems overwhelming. Consider the chapters you have read as helpful hints. That is, in fact, what they are. If a few of these ideas spark your interest and encourage you toward greater brain health, *fantastic!*

The thoughts expressed here don't come entirely from science. I wrote this book from the foundation of stewarding what God created in us. Everything else flows from the understanding that God created us as physical, emotional, and spiritual beings.

I hope we can all accept the notion that caring for ourselves is a good and worthy goal. This is a goal to be celebrated. It is not a slap on the wrist. It's not about shame or guilt. Even when we haven't been the best caretakers of some aspect of ourselves, let's leave shame out and let conviction in. Let's keep moving, even with baby steps, toward greater health.

Commencement

I love commencement ceremonies. The hearts of proud parents, relieved students, and brightly clad faculty soar to the strains of Elgar's *Pomp and Circumstance*. A festive spirit fills the field or field house during the presentation of degrees, while mothers cry. It's the end of a season of school, but mostly it's an exciting beginning. Some graduates walk away with definitive plans in hand. Others ponder, *What's next?* So much knowledge is gained during school; and finally the terrifying moment of putting that knowledge to good use arrives.

As you reach this sixtieth way to keep your brain sharp, you may contemplate where to begin. Most likely many of the 60 ways are old hat to you. But perhaps not.

Right now it might be helpful to consider which suggestions pique your interest. Do you desire to lighten your physical load by eating more healthfully? If so, let that be your first step. Or maybe you have always wondered what it's like to keep a journal to process feelings and add more meaning to your life. Perhaps you wish to fit regular outdoor walks into your weekly routine, or reach out to friends and form a book group. Whatever suggestion sparks joy in your mind, start there.

I had a wonderful etymology teacher in high school. The class involved rote memorization of a seemingly impossible volume of Greek and Latin word roots. At the beginning of the semester, Mr. Paris enthusiastically admonished us to avoid being paralyzed by the thickness of the book we would commit to memory. He jumped up and down (literally!) exclaiming, "Yard by yard, life is hard. Inch by inch, it's a cinch!" And he was right. We need a brave spirit to tackle any challenge that calls for hard work and discipline. And we need to proceed in manageable increments.

Establishing new habits often requires discipline, which isn't everyone's favorite word. But the unexpected blessing of making progress *through discipline* is to see how each positive action kindles others. You may notice that good exercise encourages better eating. If I have a soul-satisfying Pilates session followed by a nice long bike ride, I feel like drinking plenty of water and eating loads of vegetables the rest of the day. I am not tempted to "mess up" the healthful goodness of my morning by eating a bunch of junk. Good leads to better.

I hope this book will be a practical guide for you. Remember the four areas of focus that promote excellent brain health: good nutrition, regular physical activity, plenty of intellectual stimulation, and invigorating social interaction. As multifaceted individuals, we have needs in each of these realms, but let's not forget our spiritual needs as well. No matter what our view of God, the need for spiritual food is as crucial as our need for bread. Our Creator wired us this way. Let's not starve this essential part of ourselves.

As you flip back through the pages of this book, start with the low-hanging fruit. Maybe your first step toward a healthier brain is simply to rid your pantry of cheap, sugar-laden chocolate and fall in love with the high quality dark stuff. Or perhaps making a conscious effort to get more sleep would serve you best. When we are exhausted, we tend to eat poorly and let exercise lag. Whatever the greatest felt need happens to be, aim to work on that!

One more word as we venture on the path toward greater brain health. We are stronger together than we are on our own, as we learned when our youngest child ran on the high school cross-country team. At first, my husband and I thought cross-country was an individual sport. Wow, were we wrong!

Our eyes were opened to the power of teamwork at its best. As Karl-Jon and his teammates cheered for each other, they never gave up until the last runner crossed the finish line. For some, completing a race was grueling, but the beauty of faster runners coming alongside slower ones made our parental hearts burst with joy. As with any challenge, we do our best to grow and develop healthful habits when we feel support. It might be just one person, or it may be a small group of reassuring friends who come together to encourage one another in making lifestyle choices that encourage a healthier brain.

With this thought in mind, let me encourage you: You can do this! It's time to commence...for the sake of your noggin and for those who love you most.

Notes

God Made Us Smart—Let's Stay That Way

1. Anne Trafton, "The Rise and Fall of Cognitive Skills," *MIT News,* March 6, 2015, news.mit .edu/2015/brain-peaks-at-different-ages-0306.

2. Patrick J. Kiger, "Your Brain as You Age," *National Geographic,* February 28, 2016, channel .nationalgeographic.com/brain-games/articles/your-brain-as-you-age.

Chapter 1: At the Beach, Pondering Midlife Fitness

1. Dan Richards, "What Boomer Clients Fear Most," *Advisor Perspectives, Inc.*, November 7, 2016, https://www.advisorperspectives.com/articles/2016/11/07/what-boomer-clients-fear-most.

2. W.L. Xu, MD, et al, "Midlife Over-weight and Obesity Increase Late Life Dementia Risk," *Neurology,* 3 May 2011, https://www.ncbi.nlm.nih.gov/pmc/articles/PMC3100125.

Chapter 2: Take a Hike

1. Gretchen Reynolds, "How Walking in Nature Changes the Brain," *New York Times,* July 22, 2015, https://well.blogs.nytimes.com/2015/07/22/how-nature-changes-the-brain/?mcubz=3.

2. Gregory Bratman, et al., "The Benefits of Nature Experience: Improved Affect and Cognition," *Science Direct,* June 29, 2015, http://www.sciencedirect.com/science/article/pii/ S0169204615000286.

3. Vandita, "Scientific Evidence: 5 Powerful Ways Hiking Alters Your Brain," *AnonHQ.COM,* October 8, 2016, anonhq.com/scientific-evidence-5-powerful-ways-hiking-alters-brain.

4. Frances E. Kuo, "Green Play Settings Reduce ADHD Symptoms," *University of Illinois at Urbana-Champaign,* http://lhhl.illinois.edu/adhd.htm.

Chapter 3: Go Jump in the Lake

1. Lizette Borreli, "Four Brain Benefits of Swimming: Improved Blood Flow Boosts Cognitive Function, Alleviates Depression Symptoms," *Medical Daily,* October 25, 2016, http://www.medicaldaily .com/4-brain-benefits-swimming-improved-blood-flow-boosts-cognitive-function-402385.

Chapter 4: Walk It Off

1. Kirk I. Erickson, et al., "Exercise Training Increases Size of Hippocampus and Improves Memory," PNAS, January 31, 2011, http://www.pnas.org/content/108/7/3017.abstract.

2. Susan Krause Whitbourne, PhD, "Get Out and Walk, Your Brain Will Thank You," *Psychology Today,* February 15, 2011, https://www.psychologytoday.com/blog/fulfillment-any-age/201102/ get-out-and-walk-your-brain-will-thank-you.

Chapter 5: Just Keep Moving!

1. Martin Prince, et al, "The Global Prevalence of Dementia: A Systematic Review and Metaanalysis," *Alzheimer's & Dementia: The Journal of the Alzheimer's Association,* January 2013, alzheimers anddementia.com/article/S1552-5260(12)02531-9/abstract.

2. Martin Lövdén; Weili Xu, and Hui-Xin Wang, "Lifestyle Change and the Prevention of Cognitive Decline and Dementia: What is the Evidence?," *PubMed.gov,* May 26, 2013, https://www.ncbi.nlm.nih.gov/pubmed/23493129.

Chapter 6: Let's Dance

1. Anne-Marie Botek, "6 Health Benefits of Dancing," *AgingCare.com,* https://www.agingcare.com/articles/health-benefits-of-dancing-170535.htm.

2. Richard Powers, "Use It or Lose It, Dancing Makes You Smarter," *RichardPowers.com,* July 30, 2010, https://socialdance.stanford.edu/syllabi/smarter.htm.

Chapter 7: Green Thumb, Bright Mind

1. Dr. Mercola, "Why Your Brain Needs a Garden," *Mercola,* August 21, 2014, http://articles.mercola.com/sites/articles/archive/2014/08/21/gardening-impacts-brain-health.aspx.

2. Ibid.

3. Anne Harding, "Why Gardening is Good for Your Health," *CNN,* July 8, 2011, http://www.cnn.com/2011/HEALTH/07/08/why.gardening.good.

Chapter 8: Pilates…Yes, Please!

1. Danielle Thibault, "Bring Your Brain to the Game; Pilates, the Sudoku of Exercise," *Patch,* September 26, 2016, http://patch.com/new-jersey/redbank/bring-your-brain-game.

2. Kristin McGee, "Mind Your Body—Pilates for Your Brain," *Huffington Post,* December 18, 2012, http://www.huffingtonpost.com/kristin-mcgee/pilates-exercises_b_1968819.html.

Chapter 9: Nap-Time Miracles

1. Belle Beth Cooper, "How Naps Affect Your Brain and Why You Should Have One Every Day," *Buffer Social,* July 25, 2013, https://blog.bufferapp.com/how-naps-affect-your-brain-and-why-you-should-have-one-every-day.

2. Amie M. Gordon, PhD, "Your Sleep Cycle Revealed," *Psychology Today,* July 26, 2013, https://www.psychologytoday.com/blog/between-you-and-me/201307/your-sleep-cycle-revealed.

Chapter 10: "You Smoke Like Smelly the Bear"

1. Ben Spencer, "It's Never Too Late to Quit: Stubbing Out Your Habit Reverses the Harmful Effect of Smoking on the Brain and Protects Against Dementia," *Daily Mail,* 18 November 2015, http://www.dailymail.co.uk/health/article-3323879/It-s-NEVER-late-quit-Stubbing-habit-reverses-harmful-effects-smoking-brain-protects-against-dementia.html.

Chapter 11: Breathe

1. Sarah Knapton, "Take a Deep Breath…Inhaling Through Nose Stimulates Brain and Boosts Memory," *The Telegraph,* 8 December 2016, http://www.telegraph.co.uk/science/2016/12/08/take-deep-breathinhaling-nose-stimulates-brain-boosts-memory/.

Chapter 12: More Than a Helmet

1. Ester Heerema, "Preventing Alzheimer's: Can Concussions Cause Dementia?" *Very Well,* April 20, 2016, https://www.verywell.com/preventing-alzheimers-can-concussions-cause-dementia-98438.

2. Department of Health, "Traumatic Brain Injury: Prevention Is the Only Cure," *New York State Department of Health,* December 2013, https://www.health.ny.gov/publications/0660.

3. Marisa Cohen, "Protect Your Brain for Life, Follow These Expert Strategies," *Neurology Now,* February/March 2017, http://journals.lww.com/neurologynow/Fulltext/2017/13010/Protect_Your_Brain_for_Life__Follow_these_expert.19.aspx.

Chapter 13: Sleep Matters

1. Lulu Xie, et al, "Sleep Drives Metabolite Clearance from the Adult Brain," *Science,* 18 October 2013, http://science.sciencemag.org/content/342/6156/373.

2. Mark Michaud, "To Sleep, Perchance to Clean," *University of Rochester Medical Center,* October 17, 2017, https://www.urmc.rochester.edu/news/story/3956/to-sleep-perchance-to-clean.aspx.

Chapter 14: Massage: A Treat for the Mind and Body

1. Lecia Bushak, "Therapeutic Massage for Anxiety: How Touch Improves Mental Health," *Medical Daily,* August 4, 2016, http://www.medicaldaily.com/therapeutic-massage-anxiety-how-touch -therapy-improves-mental-health-393837; Dov Michaeli, MD, PhD, "Massage and Your Brain," *The Doctor Weighs In,* March 16, 2016, https://thedoctorweighsin.com/massage-and-your-brain/.

2. Alex A. Kecskeso, "Neurohormonal Effects of Massage," *Pacific College of Oriental Medicine,* November 8, 2014, http://www.pacificcollege.edu/news/blog/2014/11/08/neurohormonal-effects -massage-therapy.

3. Michaeli, "Massage and Your Brain."

4. Mayo Clinic Staff, "Massage: Get in Touch with Its Many Benefits," *Mayo Clinic,* December 7, 2015, http://www.mayoclinic.org/healthy-lifestyle/stress-management/in-depth/massage/ art-20045743.

5. Kecskeso, "Neurohormonal Effects of Massage."

Chapter 15: Popeye and Mom

1. "Healthy Eating Plate and Healthy Eating Pyramid," *Harvard School of Public Health,* 2017, https://www.hsph.harvard.edu/nutritionsource/healthy-eating-plate/.

Chapter 16: Woes of the Western Diet

1. Cynthia Ogden, "Overweight and Obesity Statistics," *National Institute of Diabetes and Digestive and Kidney Diseases,* August 2017, https://www.niddk.nih.gov/health-information/ health-statistics/overweight-obesity.

2. Michael Roizen, MD, "Food for Brain Health," *Cleveland Clinic.org,* n.d., https://my.clevelandclinic .org/ccf/media/files/Neurological_Institute/Cleveland-Clinic-Food-for-Brain-Health -Michael-Roizen.pdf.

3. Scott E. Kanoski and Terry L. Davidson, "Western Diet Consumption and Cognitive Impairment Links to Hippocampal Dysfunction and Obesity," *US National Library of Medicine,* December 16, 2010, https://www.ncbi.nlm.nih.gov/pmc/articles/PMC3056912/.

Chapter 17: Eating for Pleasure

1. Mireille Guiliano, *French Women Don't Get Fat* (New York, NY: Alfred Knopf, 2005), p. 33.

2. Fernando Gómez-Pinilla, "Brain Foods: The Effects of Nutrition on Cognition," *US National Library of Medicine,* July 9, 2008, https://www.ncbi.nlm.nih.gov/pmc/articles/PMC2805706/.

Chapter 18: The Beautiful Mediterranean Diet

1. Michael Pollan, *In Defense of Food* (New York, NY: Penguin Books, 2008), 1.

2. American Academy of Neurology "Mediterranean Diet May Have Lasting Effects on Brain Health," *Science Daily,* January 4, 2017, https://www.sciencedaily.com/releases/2017/01/170104174210 .htm.

3. Mayo Clinic Staff, "Beans and Other Legumes: Cooking Tips," *Mayo Clinic,* July 6, 2017, http://www.mayoclinic.org/healthy-lifestyle/nutrition-and-healthy-eating/in-depth/legumes/ art-20044278?pg=1.

4. Mea Hassell and Miles Hassell, MD, *Good Food Great Medicine,* Lithtex (Hillsboro, OR, 2012).

5. Diana Kelly and Sarah Klein, "Five Reasons to Eat a Handful of Nuts a Day," *Prevention,* January 6, 2016, http://www.prevention.com/health/walnuts-can-improve-your-memory.

6. Hassell and Hassell, *Good Food Great Medicine,* 5.

Chapter 19: Welcome, Omega-3s

1. Carmen Patrick Mohan, "The Facts on Omega-3 Fatty Acids," *Web MD,* May 18, 2017, http://www.webmd.com/healthy-aging/omega-3-fatty-acids-fact-sheet#1.

2. Julie Corliss, "Finding Omega-3 Fats in Fish: Farmed versus Wild," *Harvard Health Publications,* December 23, 2015, http://www.health.harvard.edu/blog/finding-omega-3-fats-in-fish-farmed -versus-wild-201512238909.

3. Tamara Duker Freuman, "How to Choose a Fish Oil Supplement," *U.S. News,* February 4, 2014, http://health.usnews.com/health-news/blogs/eat-run/2014/02/04/how-to-choose-a-fish-oil -supplement.

Chapter 20: Whole Grains

1. Rachel C. Masters, et al., "Whole and Refined Grain Intakes Are Related to Inflammatory Protein Concentrations in Human Plasma," *US National Library of Medicine,* December 17, 2009, https://www.ncbi.nlm.nih.gov/pmc/articles/PMC2821887/.

2. Hanne Risgarrd, *Home Baked* (White River Junction, VT: Chelsea Green Publishing, 2012), 34-37.

3. Richard Bertinet, *Crust* (London, England: Kyle Books, 2007), 148.

Chapter 21: Yogurt, Baby!

1. Elaine Magee, MPH, RD, "The Benefits of Yogurt," *Web MD,* March 7, 2007, http://www .webmd.com/diet/features/benefits-of-yogurt#2.

2. Eva Selhub, MD, "Nutritional Psychiatry: Your Brain on Food," *Harvard Health Publications,* November 16, 2015, http://www.health.harvard.edu/blog/nutritional-psychiatry-your-brain -on-food-201511168626.

3. Paige Vandegrift, "Homemade Yogurt," *For Love of the Table,* September 20, 2012, http://www .forloveofthetable.com/2012/09/homemade-yogurt.html.

Chapter 22: Thank Goodness for Berries

1. Tufts University Health and Nutrition Letter, "Blueberries Good for Your Blood Pressure and Brain," *Tufts University,* April 2015, http://www.nutritionletter.tufts.edu/issues/10_16/current -articles/Blueberries-Good-for-Your-Blood-Pressure-and-Brain_1690-1.html; Tufts University Health and Nutrition Letter, "Pick Berries to Protect Your Aging Brain," *Tufts University,* July 2012, http://www.nutritionletter.tufts.edu/issues/8_7/current-articles/Pick-Berries-to-Protect -Your-Aging-Brain_877-1.html.

2. Michael Murray, *The Encyclopedia of Healing Foods* (New York, NY: Atria Books, 2005), 314.

3. Ibid., 312.

4. Jessica Maki, "Berries Keep Your Brain Sharp," *Harvard Gazette,* April 26, 2012, http://news .harvard.edu/gazette/story/2012/04/berries-keep-your-brain-sharp/.

Chapter 23: Java—for Goodness Sake

1. Latarsha Gatlin, "Caffeine Has Positive Effect on Memory, Johns Hopkins Researchers Say," *John Hopkins University,* January 12, 2014, http://hub.jhu.edu/2014/01/12/caffeine-enhances -memory/.

2. Lecia Bushak, "Health Benefits of Coffee: Caffeine Acts as an Antioxidant, Fights Free Radicals," *Medical Daily*, May 4, 2015, http://www.medicaldaily.com/health-benefits-coffee-caffeine-acts-antioxidant-fights-free-radicals-331856.

3. Galtin, "Caffeine Has Positive Effect on Memory."

Chapter 24: Healthful Hydration

1. Markham Heid, "Your Brain on Dehydration," *Shape*, 2017, http://www.shape.com/lifestyle/mind-and-body/your-brain-dehydration.

2. Melinda Johnson, "Tips on Hydration from Sports Dietitians," *U.S. News.*, July 19, 2013, http://health.usnews.com/health-news/blogs/eat-run/2013/07/19/tips-on-hydration-from-sports-dietitians.

3. Nsikan Akpan, "Stay Hydrated, Stay Smart: Quenching Thirst with Water Boosts Brain Power," *Medical Daily*, July 16, 2013, http://www.medicaldaily.com/stay-hydrated-stay-smart-quenching-thirst-water-boosts-brain-power-247723.

4. Heid, "Your Brain on Dehydration."

5. Akpan, "Stay Hydrated, Stay Smart."

6. Johnson, "Tips on Hydration from Sports Dieticians."

Chapter 25: Chocolate on the Brain

1. Roberto A. Ferdman, "The Magical Thing Eating Chocolate Does to Your Brain," *The Washington Post*, March 4, 2016, https://www.washingtonpost.com/news/wonk/wp/2016/03/04/the-magical-thing-eating-chocolate-does-to-your-brain/?utm_term=.9a69ad81463e.

2. Ferdman, "The Magical Thing Eating Chocolate Does"; Deane Alban, "9 Brain Boosting Benefits of Dark Chocolate," *Be Brain Fit*, February 2017, https://bebrainfit.com/brain-benefits-dark-chocolate/.

3. Alban, "9 Brain Boosting Benefits"; Alice G. Walton, "Cognition Link Gives One More Reason to Eat Chocolate," *Forbes*, February 24, 2016, http://www.forbes.com/sites/alicegwalton/2016/02/24/the-chocolate-cognition-connection/#7610befb6167.

4. Heidi Godman, "Cocoa: A Sweet Treat for the Brain," *Harvard Health Publications*, October 29, 2015, http://www.health.harvard.edu/blog/cocoa-sweet-treat-brain-201502057676.

5. Alban, "Cognition Link Gives One More Reason to Eat Chocolate."

6. Deena Shanker, *Grist*, February 13, 2013, "A Guide To Ethical Chocolate," http://grist.org/food/a-guide-to-ethical-chocolate.

Chapter 26: Why Dad Should Move to Minnesota

1. Cody C. Delistraty, "The Importance of Eating Together," *The Atlantic*, July 18, 2014, https://www.theatlantic.com/health/archive/2014/07/the-importance-of-eating-together/374256/.

2. Ibid.

3. "Eating Alone Unhealthy for the Elderly," WebMD, 1999, http://www.webmd.com/healthy-aging/news/19991015/eating-alone-unhealthy-for-elderly-news#2.

4. Annalijn Conklin, "Meals for One: Eating Alone Unhealthy for the Elderly," *University of Cambridge*, 19 October 2013, http://www.cam.ac.uk/research/discussion/meals-for-one-how-eating-alone-affects-the-health-of-the-elderly.

5. Ibid.

Chapter 27: Brain Games

1. Sandra Bond Chapman, et al, "Neural Mechanisms of Brain Plasticity with Complex Cognitive Training in Healthy Seniors," *US National Library of Medicine,* 28 August 2013, https://www.ncbi.nlm.nih.gov/pmc/articles/PMC4351428/.

2. Melissa Malamut, "How To Improve Your Brain Health," *Boston,* October 5, 2012, http://www.bostonmagazine.com/health/blog/2012/10/05/improve-brain-health-decrease-risk-dementia/.

3. ST Cheng, AC Chan, and EC Yu, "An Exploratory Study of the Effect of Mahjonj on the Cognitive Function of Persons with Dementia," *US National Library of Health,* 21 July 2006, https://www.ncbi.nlm.nih.gov/pubmed/16779765.

Chapter 29: No Pain, No Gain!

1. Lauren Silverman, "Learning a New Skill Works Best to Keep Your Brain Sharp," *National Public Radio,* May 5, 2014, http://www.npr.org/sections/health-shots/2014/05/05/309006780/learning-a-new-skill-works-best-to-keep-your-brain-sharp.

Chapter 30: In Favor of Memorizing

1. Radiological Society of North America, "Rote Learning Improves Memory in Seniors," *Science Daily,* November 29, 2006, www.sciencedaily.com/releases/2006/11/061128084444.htm.

Chapter 31: Music's Mind-Boggling Benefits

1. Catherine Y. Wan and Gotfried Schlaug, "Music Making as a Tool for Promoting Brain Plasticity Across the Lifespan," *US National Library of Medicine,* 16 October 2010, https://www.ncbi.nlm.nih.gov/pmc/articles/PMC2996135/.

2. Ibid.

Chapter 32: Journaling Observed

1. Adaline Bjorkman, *While It Was Still Dark* (Chicago, IL: Covenant Press, 1978), vi-viii.

2. Stuart Wolpert, "Putting Feelings into Words Produces Therapeutic Effects in the Brain; UCLA Neuroimaging Study Supports Ancient Buddhist Teachings," *UCLA Newsroom,* June 21, 2007, http://newsroom.ucla.edu/releases/Putting-Feelings-Into-Words-Produces-8047.

3. Kristen Clark, "Journaling Through Your Emotions," His Side of the Looking Glass, n.d., http://hissideofthelookingglass.com/journaling-through-your-emotions/.

4. Thai Nguyen, "10 Surprising Benefits You'll Get from Keeping a Journal," *Huff Post,* February 13, 2015, http://www.huffingtonpost.com/thai-nguyen/benefits-of-journaling-_b_6648884.html.

5. Ibid.

6. Ibid.

7. Ibid.

Chapter 33: On Being Bilingual

1. Tanya Lewis, "Bilingual People Are like Brain 'Bodybuilders," *Live Science,* November 12, 2014, http://www.livescience.com/48721-bilingual-brain-bodybuilders.html.

2. Mia Nacamulli, "The Benefits of the Bilingual Brain," *TED Ed,* June 2, 2015, https://ed.ted.com/lessons/how-speaking-multiple-languages-benefits-the-brain-mia-nacamulli.

3. Harrison Wein, PhD, "Bilingual Effects in the Brain," *National Institutes of Health,* May 7, 2012, https://www.nih.gov/news-events/nih-research-matters/bilingual-effects-brain.

Chapter 34: Art and Arteries

1. Angela Clow, PhD and Catherine Fredhoi, MSc, "Normalisation of Salivary Cortisol Levels and Self-Report Stress by a Brief Lunchtime Visit to an Art Gallery by London City Workers," *Research Gate,* January 2006, https://www.researchgate.net/publication/252281628_ Normalisation_of_salivary_cortisol_levels_and_self-report_stress_by_a_brief_lunchtime_visit _to_an_art_gallery_by_London_City_workers.

2. Gabe Bergado, "Science Shows Art Can Do Incredible Things for Your Mind and Body," *Mic,* December 15, 2014, https://mic.com/articles/106504/science-shows-that-art-is-having-fantastic -effects-on-our-brains-and-bodies#.lvZkK3Sta.

Chapter 35: Creating Art

1. Barbara Bagan, PhD, "Aging, What's Art Got to Do with It?" *Today's Geriatric Medicine,* n.d., http://www.todaysgeriatricmedicine.com/news/ex_082809_03.shtml; Gabe Bergado, "Science Shows Art Can Do Incredible Things for Your Mind and Body," *Mic,* December 15, 2014, https://mic.com/articles/106504/science-shows-that-art-is-having-fantastic-effects-on-our -brains-and-bodies#.45mQeamIz.

2. Anne Bolwerk, Jessica Mack-Andrick, et al. "How Art Changes Your Brain: Differential Effects of Visual Art Production and Cognitive Art Evaluation on Functional Brain Connectivity," *PLOS,* July 1, 2014, http://journals.plos.org/plosone/article?id=10.1371/journal.pone.0101035.

Chapter 36: You've Got Mail!

1. Diana Raab, "Six Reasons Why Letter Writing Is Good for Your Mind and Your Body," *Brain Speak,* n.d., http://brainspeak.com/6-reasons-letter-writing-good-mind-body/.

2. Alena Hall, "Nine Reasons to Not Abandon the Art of the Handwritten Letter," *Huff Post,* January 11, 2015, http://www.huffingtonpost.com/2015/01/11/benefits-of-writing-letters-and -postcards_n_6425540.html.

3. Yohanna Desta, "Seven Ways Writing by Hand Can Save Your Brain," *Mashable,* January 19, 2015, http://mashable.com/2015/01/19/handwriting-brain-benefits/#h6rv5joFzsqw.

Chapter 37: Learning for a Lifetime

1. Kathryn Doyle, PhD, "Keeping the Aging Brain Active May Also Keep It Sharp: Study," *Reuters,* June 23, 2014, http://www.reuters.com/article/us-cognitive-activity-dementia-idUSKBN 0EY2KU20140623.

2. Romeo Vitelli, "Can Lifelong Learning Help as We Age?" *Psychology Today,* October 14, 2012, https://www.psychologytoday.com/blog/media-spotlight/201210/can-lifelong-learning -help-we-age.

3. Nancy Nordenson, *Just Think* (Grand Rapids, MI: Baker Books, 2003), 141-151.

Chapter 38: What's So Special About Poetry?

1. Richard Alleyne, "Writing Poems Helps Brain Cope with Turmoil, Say Scientists," *The Telegraph,* 15 February 2009, http://www.telegraph.co.uk/culture/culturenews/4630043/AAAS-Writing -poems-helps-brain-cope-with-emotional-turmoil-say-scientists.html.

2. Ibid.

3. University Staff, "Poetry Is like Music to the Mind, Scientists Prove," *University of Exeter,* 9 October 2013, http://www.exeter.ac.uk/news/featurednews/title_324631_en.html.

4. "Poetry, Music, Emotions and the Brain," *British Council,* n.d., http://learnenglishteens.british council.org/uk-now/science-uk/poetry-music-emotions-and-brain.

Chapter 39: Laughter: Still the Best Medicine

1. Anne Francis, "Laughter Improves Brain Work, Good for Short Term Memory," *TechTimes*, 23 April 2014, http://www.techtimes.com/articles/5898/20140423/laughter-improves-brain-work -good-for-short-term-memory.htm.

2. Thomas Crook, PhD, "This Is Your Brain on Laughter," *Prevention*, November 3, 2011, http:// www.prevention.com/health/brain-health/your-brain-laughter.

3. Ibid.

Chapter 40: Any Volunteers?

1. Stephanie Watson, "Volunteering May Be Good for Body and Mind," *Harvard Health Publications*, June 26, 2013, http://www.health.harvard.edu/blog/volunteering-may-be-good -for-body-and-mind-201306266428.

2. Robert Grimm Jr., et al, "The Health Benefits of Volunteering," *National & Community Service*, April 2007, https://www.nationalservice.gov/pdf/07_0506_hbr.pdf.

Chapter 41: From Zippers to Chickadees

1. Jordan E. Rosenfeld, "These Young People Are Helping Older Adults Stay Current with Technology," *Alternet*, July 13, 2015, http://www.alternet.org/education/these-young-people-are -helping-older-adults-stay-current-technology.

2. Jean Rhodes, "Mentoring Youth Promotes Cognitive Gains in Older Adults," *The Chronicle*, October 28, 2013, http://chronicle.umbmentoring.org/mentoring-youth-promotes-cognitive -gains-in-older-adults/.

Chapter 42: Choral Singing for the Health of It

1. Stephen Clift, et al, "Choral Singing, Wellbeing and Health: Summary of Findings from a Cross-National Survey," *Canterbury Christ Church University*, 2008, https://www.canterbury .ac.uk/health-and-wellbeing/sidney-de-haan-research-centre/documents/choral-singing- summary-report.pdf.

2. Fiona Macrae, "Why Singing Is the Fast Way to Friendship: Chemicals Released from the Brain Help Us Bond Quickly," *Daily Mail*, 27 Ocotber 2015, http://www.dailymail.co.uk/news/ article-3292784/Why-singing-fast-way-friendship-Chemicals-released-brain-helps-people -bond-quickly-group-activities.html.

3. Ibid.

4. Ibid.

Chapter 44: Book Group: More Than a Good Read

1. Dr. Michael Roizen, "How Can Joining a Book Club Improve My Health?" *Share Care*, n.d., https://www.sharecare.com/health/healthy-habits/how-book-club-improve-health.

2. Delia Lloyd, "Five Reasons to Join a Book Club," *HuffPost*, May 25, 2011, http://www.huffington post.com/delia-lloyd/five-reasons-to-join-a-bo_b_476162.html.

Chapter 45: One Thing at a Time

1. Deane Alban, "The Cognitive Cost of Multitasking," *Be Brain Fit*, 20 April 2017, https:// bebrainfit.com/cognitive-costs-multitasking/.

2. Ibid.

3. Ibid.

4. Ibid.

5. Ibid.

6. Patrick J. Skerrett, "Multitasking—A Medical and Mental Hazard," *Harvard Health Publications*, January 7, 2012, http://www.health.harvard.edu/blog/multitasking-a-medical-and-mental-hazard-201201074063.

7. Chris Woolston, "Multitasking and Stress," *HealthDay*, January 20, 2017, https://consumer.healthday.com/encyclopedia/emotional-health-17/emotional-disorder-news-228/multitasking-and-stress-646052.html.

8. Skerrett, "Multitasking and Stress."

Chapter 46: Pets—Best Friends with Benefits

1. Sy Montgomery, "Psychological Effects of Pets are Profound," *Boston Globe*, January 12, 2015, https://www.bostonglobe.com/lifestyle/2015/01/12/your-brain-pets/geoJHAfFHxrwNS4OgWb7sO/story.html.

2. Stanley Coren, PhD, "Health and Psychological Benefits of Bonding with a Pet Dog," *Psychology Today*, June 7, 2009, https://www.psychologytoday.com/blog/canine-corner/200906/health-and-psychological-benefits-bonding-pet-dog.

3. Andrea Beetz, "Psychosocial and Psychophysiological Effects of Human-Animal Interactions: The Possible Role of Oxytocin," *US National Library of Medicine*, 9 July 2012, https://www.ncbi.nlm.nih.gov/pmc/articles/PMC3408111/.

Chapter 48: Grateful Heart, Peaceful Mind

1. Christian Jarrett, "How Expressing Gratitude Might Change Your Brain," *New York*, January 7, 2016, http://nymag.com/scienceofus/2016/01/how-expressing-gratitude-change-your-brain.html.

2. Harvard Medical Letter, "In Praise of Gratitude," *Harvard Health Publications*, November 2011, http://www.health.harvard.edu/newsletter_article/in-praise-of-gratitude.

3. Ibid.

Chapter 49: Relationships of the Grandest Kind

1. Sara M. Moorman, PhD and Jeffrey E. Stokes, MA, "Solidarity in the Grandparent–Adult Grandchild Relationship and Trajectories of Depressive Symptoms," *OxfordAcademic*, 6 June 2014, https://academic.oup.com/gerontologist/article/56/3/408/2605571/Solidarity-in-the-Grandparent-Adult-Grandchild.

Chapter 50: Mindfulness and the Man with the Yellow Hat

1. Christina Congleton, Britta K. Hözel, and Sara W. Lazar, "Mindfulness Can Literally Change Your Brain," *Harvard Business Review*, January 8, 2015, https://hbr.org/2015/01/mindfulness-can-literally-change-your-brain.

2. Jennifer Wolkin, "How the Brain Changes When You Meditate," *Mindful*, September 20, 2015, http://www.mindful.org/how-the-brain-changes-when-you-meditate/.

Chapter 51: Mind the Good Stuff

1. Kevin Tupper, "Christian Mindfulness," *Christian Simplicity*, n.d., http://christiansimplicity.com/christian-mindfulness/; Kelle Walsh, "Mindfulness Supports Wise Indulgence," http://www.mindful.org/mindfulness-supports-wise-indulgence/.

Chapter 54: Choosing to Be Brave

1. Kathryn Doyle, "Keeping the Aging Brain Active May Also Keep It Sharp," *Reuters*, June 23, 2014, http://www.reuters.com/article/us-cognitive-activity-dementia-idUSKBN0EY2KU20140623.

Chapter 56: Free to Forgive, Forgive to Be Free

1. Mayo Clinic Staff, "Forgiveness; Letting Go of Grudges and Bitterness," *Mayo Clinic,* November 11, 2014, http://www.mayoclinic.org/healthy-lifestyle/adult-health/in-depth/art-20047692.

2. Everett L. Worthington Jr., "The New Science of Forgiveness," *Greater Good Magazine,* September 1, 2004, http://greatergood.berkeley.edu/article/item/the_new_science_of_forgiveness.

3. "Forgiveness:YourHealthDependsonIt,"*JohnsHopkinsMedicine,*n.d.,http://www.hopkinsmedicine.org/health/healthy_aging/healthy_connections/forgiveness-your-health-depends-on-it.

4. Worthington, "The New Science of Foregiveness."

5. Jeremy Adam Smith, "Forgiveness in Action," *Greater Good Magazine,* January 31, 2007, http://greatergood.berkeley.edu/article/item/forgiveness_in_action.

6. Worthington, "The New Science of Forgiveness."

7. Emiliano Ricciardi, et al., "How the Brain Heals Emotional Wounds: The Functional Neuroanatomy of Forgiveness," *US National Library of Medicine,* 9 December 2013, https://www.ncbi.nlm.nih.gov/pmc/articles/PMC3856773/.

8. Lecia Bushak, "How Forgiveness Benefits Your Health: Forgiving Wrongdoers Can Expand Physical Fitness," *Medical Daily,* January 7, 2015, http://www.medicaldaily.com/how-forgiveness-benefits-your-health-forgiving-wrongdoers-can-expand-physical-fitness-316902.

Chapter 57: Conversations with God

1. Robert Crosby, "Faith and the Brain," *Christianity Today,* Summer 2014, http://www.christianitytoday.com/pastors/2014/summer/faith-and-brain.html.

2. Ibid.

Chapter 58: Drinking from the Half-Full Cup

1. Mayo Clinic Staff, "Positive Thinking, Stop Negative Self-talk to Reduce Stress," *Mayo Clinic,* February 18, 2017, http://www.mayoclinic.org/healthy-lifestyle/stress-management/in-depth/positive-thinking/art-20043950.

2. Teresa Aubele, PhD and Susan Reynolds, "Happy Brain, Happy Life," *Psychology Today,* August 2, 2011, https://www.psychologytoday.com/blog/prime-your-gray-cells/201108/happy-brain-happy-life.

3. Linda J. Solie, PhD, *Take Charge of Your Emotions* (Minneapolis, MN: Bethany House, 2013), 35-51.

About the Author

Bonnie Sparrman is a registered nurse who started her career in home-health nursing. She loved her patients throughout a wide swath of Western Michigan as well as the autonomy of home care. With the advent of her own family, Bonnie came back to the hospital in obstetrics, where she enjoyed caring for mothers and their newborns. She taught childbirth and parenting classes for nearly ten years in Michigan, northern Virginia, and Kansas City.

Still, cooking and writing have been first loves, and eventually days in the hospital were traded for teaching culinary classes, leading corporate team-building sessions, and working on books. Bonnie is the author of two books written to inspire mothers.

Bonnie and her husband, Eric, have three young-adult children of their own—Johanna, Bjorn, and Karl-Jon—and claim Isabel, their German exchange student, as a bonus daughter.

In her free time, Bonnie loves to cook, bake, welcome guests, read, hike, swim, and cycle. She prefers being outdoors in nature and loves to ride her bike with Eric, her favorite biking buddy. Together they take to the trails that encircle the lovely Minneapolis lakes near their home. Bonnie never rides faster than when she's off to mail a letter at their local post office.